Diabetes in Focus

Diabetes in Focus

Second edition

Anjana Patel

BPharm, MSc, PhD, MRPharmS

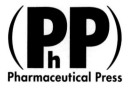

London • Chicago **Pharmaceutical Press**

Published by the Pharmaceutical Press
Publications division of the Royal Pharmaceutical Society of
Great Britain

1 Lambeth High Street, London SE1 7JN, UK
100 South Atkinson Road, Suite 206, Grayslake,
IL 60030-7820, USA

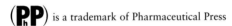 is a trademark of Pharmaceutical Press

First edition published 1999
Second edition published 2003

Text design by Barker/Hilsdon, Lyme Regis, Dorset
Typeset by Type Study, Scarborough, North Yorkshire
Printed in Great Britain by TJ International, Padstow, Cornwall

ISBN 0 85369 505 9

A catalogue record for this book is available from the British Library

The cover design shows details of the islets of Langerhans

Understanding inevitably leads to hope

Contents

Preface

This book is about the practical pharmaceutical care that pharmacists can provide for people with diabetes mellitus. The concept of collaborative pharmaceutical care has been defined and adopted by the *International Pharmaceutical Federation (FIP)* and the *World Medical Association (WMA)* as the result of the 1998 Pharmacy World Congress '*Building bridges for the benefit of the patient*'. The purpose of the policy statement on pharmaceutical care is to provide a world-wide acceptable definition of pharmaceutical care and the requirements for its implementation and practice principles. Pharmaceutical care has been defined by the FIP as being '. . . *the responsible provision of pharmacotherapy for the purpose of achieving definite outcomes that improve or maintain a patient's quality of life. It is a collaborative process that aims to prevent or identify and solve medicinal product and health related problems. This is a continuous quality improvement process for the use of medicinal products*'. The emphasis of the joint statement by the FIP and WMA on the working relationships between pharmacists and doctors in medicinal therapy is on the complementary nature and supportive responsibilities of the two professions for achieving optimal medicinal therapy for the patient. Even though there appears to be some confusion in the UK about the differences between the concepts of pharmaceutical care and medicines management, the concept of patient-centred care provided by a team of healthcare professionals is now widely accepted. The Department of Health's National Service Framework for Diabetes has acknowledged the central role that pharmacists can play in improving medicines management in people with diabetes, both in the capacity of a regular point of contact and as supplementary prescribers for chronic conditions such as diabetes. Guidance on medicines management for diabetes is being developed along the same lines as guidance produced as a part of the National Service Framework for older people.

The definition of pharmaceutical care adopted for this book includes the concept of medication assessments carried out by a pharmacist. The aim of the pharmaceutical assessment is to ensure that all medication taken by people with diabetes is effective, safe and convenient for an individual person with diabetes. It is assumed that these pharmaceutical assessments will require the development of care plans in order to identify, resolve and prevent problems with drug therapy and enable the process of supporting people with diabetes to achieve therapeutic targets. Although the cost-effectiveness of therapeutic management of diabetes is an important challenge facing the healthcare providers, this aspect is considered to be beyond the scope of this book.

Drug therapy, when used in combination with dietary and lifestyle management, forms a major component of diabetes management. Pharmacists can make a significant contribution toward the healthcare of people with diabetes through provision of information not only on drug therapy but also on lifestyle measures which help to prevent diabetic complications. The concept of pharmacists providing drug information on prescribed medication and 'over-the-counter' (OTC) products is not new. However, traditionally, pharmaceutical services have been product-orientated rather than patient-orientated because the pharmacist has mainly been involved in ensuring the quality and the accuracy of supply of the pharmaceutical product. This has meant providing general drug information and generic 'patient counselling' such as: 'What is the medication?'; 'When should the medication be taken?'; 'How should the medication be taken?'; and 'How should the medication be stored?'. The new challenge for pharmacists, outlined by the Royal Pharmaceutical Society's *'Pharmacy in the New Age'* initiative, is to extend this role and adopt a patient-centred, evidence-based approach to the delivery of comprehensive pharmaceutical care. The fundamental requirement for this type of approach is the formation of collaborative relationships between the pharmacist, the patient and other healthcare professionals involved in the care of the patient. This is in line with the patient-orientated team approach advocated for the effective management of diabetes mellitus.

Pharmacy is a scientific discipline, whereas the delivery of pharmaceutical care is partly a vocational undertaking. In order to provide comprehensive pharmaceutical care, pharmacists require information which is both accessible and relevant to the situation of the patient. This book has been written with the information needs of the pharmacist in mind. All too often the scientific and clinical aspects of drug therapy are divorced. The aim of this book is to combine the two aspects and to present scientific information in the context of clinical practice. The book provides a summary of information currently available on diabetes management, particularly in relation to drug therapy. Information has been drawn from a wide range of published sources and is structured to highlight the currently available national and international guidelines on diabetes management including the National Service Framework for Diabetes and the National Institute for Clinical Excellence clinical guidelines for the management of type 2 diabetes.

Individual chapters provide concise overviews of the different aspects of diabetes mellitus and its management. In order to aid practical application of the information contained within this book, a series of 'Focus Points' have been highlighted throughout the text. The purpose of these 'Focus points' is to provide brief summaries or overviews of key aspects of diabetes management including Adverse Effects, Diagnostic, Glucose Monitoring, Glycaemic Control, Insulin Dosage, Management, Risk Factors and Screening Factors. The information contained within the 'Focus Point' boxes can be used both in the context of individual chapters or separately as an *aide-mémoire*.

The introductory chapter provides an overview of the challenges of diabetes mellitus management. Chapter 2 covers the World Health Organization classification and diagnostic criteria for diabetes mellitus, while Chapter 3 provides an overview of factors that affect development of diabetic complications and some basic principles for management. Chapter 4 is devoted to the key principles of lifestyle management that can have a major impact on daily lives of people with diabetes, and Chapter 5 covers major aspects of monitoring glycaemic control. Chapter 6 provides an overview of the dietary recommendations, and Chapter 7 summarises the pharmacological principles and the clinical rationale underpinning the current approaches for type 2 diabetes management. Chapters 8 to 13 provide therapeutics monographs for different classes of pharmacotherapeutic interventions including insulins, sulphonylureas, metformin, acarbose, thiazolidinediones (PPAR-γ-agonists) and meglitinides. Chapter 14 provides a brief overview of new therapies currently being investigated for diabetes management. Chapter 15 covers population screening for early identification of people with type 2 diabetes, and Chapter 16 is devoted to the pharmaceutical assessment of people with diabetes and provides practical 'checklists' which pharmacists can use to minimise the risks of the disease and treatment in people with diabetes.

It is beyond the scope of this book to cover specialist aspects of diabetes care required during childhood, pregnancy or surgery. Similarly, it has not been possible to cover comprehensively the non-drug aspects of diabetes care such as patient education and psychological care. For further information, please see the summary of the evidence base for the key recommendations from the National Service Framework for Diabetes Standards (2002) for adults with type 2 diabetes, and the list of Useful Resources, both of which are provided at the end of the book.

It is hoped that the format of the book will enable pharmacists – regardless of their level of expertise – to gain access to the information necessary for providing effective pharmaceutical care for people with diabetes. The field of diabetes is rapidly expanding, and within the past few years there has been an explosion of information available on the subject. While every effort has been made to check the accuracy of the information contained within the book, the rapidly changing nature of the subject matter must be borne in mind during its use. This is particularly important where drug dosages and adverse effects are concerned. Consultation of the most recent version of the manufacturer's drug data sheet or SPC (specification of product characteristics) to validate the drug dosage information is recommended.

Diabetes mellitus presents the pharmacist with major opportunities to provide effective pharmaceutical care. This book provides the information basis for the development of pharmaceutical care for people with diabetes.

Acknowledgements

My sincere thanks are due to the people of the South Asian community living with diabetes. Their willingness to share their experiences made it possible for me to focus on the practical aspects of pharmaceutical care.

My thanks are also due to John Sampson for providing the index and to staff at Pharmaceutical Press for their input into the manuscript.

About the author

Anjana Patel is a pharmacist with a special interest in diabetes. She is also interested in promoting evidence-based practice through effective dissemination of high-quality validated information to 'front-line' healthcare professionals.

Anjana graduated in 1980 from Chelsea College, University of London (BPharm Hons) and completed her pre-registration in Community Pharmacy. Following a year working as a Community Pharmacist, Anjana joined the pharmacy department at St Thomas' Hospital, London, where she worked from 1982 to 1987, obtaining an MSc in pharmacology and holding the position of Staff Pharmacist. Anjana then spent 3 years at the Welsh School of Pharmacy undertaking full-time research, and in 1990 obtained her PhD in the medicinal chemistry of enkephalinase enzyme inhibitors. Between 1990 and 1996, Anjana was based at the Royal Pharmaceutical Society of Great Britain as Assistant Editor, *British National Formulary* (BNF). Between 1996 and 2001, she worked as an independent pharmaceutical consultant in primary care, during which time her range of projects included improving collaborative working practices between Community Pharmacists and GPs and the development of an effective secondary–primary care interface for the communication of patient medication information from hospitals to GPs. Anjana has been a Clinical Editor of *BMJ Clinical Evidence* since April 2001. Her current interests include exploring ways to identify, process and present evidence relating to the harms of therapeutic interventions, and the role of traditional herbal medicines in an allopathic medical system. Her other publications include chapters on enzyme inhibitors and a book on the community history of Leva Patidar Patels of Charotar.

The views expressed in this book are those of the author and do not necessarily correspond to those of *BMJ Clinical Evidence*.

Focus points

1

Introduction

Diabetes mellitus is a common chronic disorder and represents a serious healthcare challenge. It greatly increases the risk of coronary heart disease and stroke, and is a leading cause of blindness, kidney failure and limb amputations. The prevalence of diabetes is on the increase, and an estimated 239 million people world-wide are expected to have the condition by the year 2020. This is reflected in the increased incidence of both type 1 and type 2 diabetes in the UK. In 1995, it was estimated that about 1 380 000 adults had confirmed diabetes mellitus, since when it has been estimated that about 1 000 000 people have diabetes which has not been diagnosed.[1] The prevalence of diabetes increases with age. One in twenty people in the UK over the age of 65 years have type 2 diabetes, and this increases to one in five people over the age of 85 years.[2]

The reasons for the increase in type 1 diabetes is still unclear. Although identification of genes that predispose both children and adults to type 1 diabetes has progressed considerably, the evidence for environmental trigger factors remains unclear. However there is strong consensus that the increase in type 1 diabetes is more likely to be linked to environmental factors rather than genetic ones. The factors influencing the increase in type 2 diabetes are complex and, as yet, not fully understood. Nonetheless, these factors are likely to include an increase in the number of people at risk of developing type 2 diabetes due to the decline in physical activity and an increase in dietary energy intake, an increase in survival of people with type 2 diabetes, and an increase in detection of previously undiagnosed type 2 diabetes. Early detection of type 2 diabetes is a key factor in preventing the development of diabetic complications. There is now some good evidence that changes in lifestyle may help to delay and possibly prevent the onset of type 2 diabetes.[3]

Considerable progress has been made in the understanding of diabetes management since the targets for diabetes care were set by the *St Vincent Declaration* under the aegis of the European sections of the *World Health Organization* (WHO) and the *International Diabetes*

Federation.[1] These targets represented a turning point in the approach to healthcare of people with diabetes mellitus. The main target is to improve both the quality and duration of life and to encourage people with diabetes to take responsibility for their illness and to achieve independence in the management of their condition. Teamwork and collaboration are essential components of successful diabetes management.

Diabetes mellitus is a life-long condition, and people diagnosed with the condition require considerable support from healthcare professionals – particularly at the time of initial diagnosis and when complications of diabetes require treatment. For people with type 1 diabetes, the development of quick-acting insulin analogues (insulin lispro, insulin aspart) and a long-acting insulin analogue (insulin glargine), have provided the possibility of tailoring insulin regimens to individual lifestyle as alternatives to strict daily diet and insulin-injecting regimens. For people with type 2 diabetes, it is now also recognised that effective management involves much more than achieving moderate glycaemic control. Evidence from large clinical trials has indicated that significant improvement in cardiovascular outcome can be achieved by tight control of risk factors such as hypertension, hyperglycaemia and dyslipidaemia in people with type 2 diabetes. This has resulted in the setting of ambitious targets for risk factor control with therapeutic interventions. However, the therapeutic regimens needed for tight control of several risk factors at the same time has resulted in polypharmacy for many people with type 2 diabetes.[4] A further complicating factor is that a large proportion of people with type 2 diabetes tend to be elderly and are the most vulnerable to adverse effects of therapeutic drugs, particularly where there is polypharmacy. On the other hand, the diagnosis of diabetes may be delayed in elderly people because of symptoms being wrongly attributed to effects of aging.[2]

The provision of diabetes services is complex, as care is provided by a wide range of healthcare professionals including specialist diabetes teams, general practitioners (GPs), community health staff, people with diabetes themselves and their carers. Elderly people with diabetes tend to have complex needs requiring multidisciplinary care, requiring co-ordination across primary, secondary and residential care and social services. The provision of information, education and support for elderly people with diabetes can have a major impact on effectiveness of diabetes management.[2]

References

1. Diabetes in the United Kingdom – 1996. A British Diabetic Association Report. www.diabetes.org.uk (last accessed December 2002).
2. Department of Health. National Service Framework for Diabetes: Standards 2002. Additional material: Health Inequalities. www.doh.gov.uk/nsf/diabetes (last accessed November 2002).
3. New hope for Type 2 diabetes prevention. Diabetes Update. Autumn 2001. www.diabetes.org.uk (last accessed December 2002).
4. Emslie-Smith A, Dowell J, Morris A. The problem of polypharmacy in type 2 diabetes. *Br J Diabetes Vasc Dis* 2003; 3: 54–56.

2

The diabetic syndrome

Diabetes mellitus is a chronic and progressive disease which can affect people in all age groups and can cause ill health, disability and premature death. It is a heterogeneous disorder characterised by varying degrees of insulin resistance and insulin deficiency, which lead to a disturbance in glucose homeostasis. In the short term, uncontrolled diabetes is characterised by symptoms of high blood glucose levels (hyperglycaemia). Patients with mild hyperglycaemia do not usually experience any symptoms and therefore may be unaware that they have diabetes for several years. Symptoms of marked hyperglycaemia include thirst (polydipsia), large volume of urine (polyuria), frequent feeling of hunger (polyphagia), feeling of tiredness, blurred vision, and weight gain or weight loss. Acute life-threatening consequences of untreated diabetes mellitus include hyperglycaemia with ketoacidosis (see pp. 33–34) or non-ketotic hyperosmolar coma (see pp. 34–35). In the long term, people with diabetes are predisposed to cardiovascular, peripheral vascular and cerebrovascular disease, as well as microvascular complications leading to retinopathy, nephropathy or neuropathy with an increase in risk of foot ulcers and amputation (see Chapter 3).[1-4]

WHO diagnostic criteria

The World Health Organization (WHO) has revised its 'Definition, Diagnosis and Classification of Diabetes Mellitus and its Complications'.[4] Diabetes UK (formerly known as the British Diabetic Association) has recommended that all UK health professionals adopt the new criteria from 1st June 2000. The revised criteria have also been endorsed by the Department of Health.[5,6]

Criteria for people presenting with symptoms of diabetes

- Symptoms of diabetes (polyuria, polydipsia and unexplained weight loss) *PLUS*

- A random venous plasma glucose concentration ≥11.1 mmol/L (whole blood ≥9.5 mmol/L)
- *OR* a fasting venous plasma glucose concentration ≥7.0 mmol/L (whole blood ≥6.1 mmol/L)
- *OR* a venous plasma glucose concentration ≥11.1 mmol/L at 2 h after 75 g anhydrous glucose in an oral glucose tolerance test (OGTT).

Criteria for people who are asymptomatic

- If blood glucose levels outside normal range with a self-monitoring 'stick' test (whole blood), confirm blood glucose levels with venous plasma determination *PLUS*
- At least one additional glucose test (fasting, random, or 2-h post glucose load OGTT; see Diagnostic Focus, below) carried out on a separate day with a value in the diagnostic diabetic range essential for diagnosis for diabetes mellitus.

Criteria for people who have high blood glucose but less than diabetic range

The WHO have now defined two categories of impaired glucose regulation for people who have blood glucose levels which are above the normal range but are not in the diabetic range.

- Impaired glucose tolerance (IGT) is defined as fasting venous plasma glucose <7.0 mmol/L with an OGTT (see Diagnostic Focus, below) test 2-h value between 7.8 mmol and 11.1 mmol/L. Impaired glucose tolerance is considered to be a risk category for cardiovascular disease.
- Impaired fasting glycaemia (IFG) is defined as fasting venous plasma glucose value between 6.1 and 7.0 mmol/L). IFG is considered to be a risk

DIAGNOSTIC FOCUS

Oral glucose tolerance test (OGTT)

The oral glucose tolerance test (*2-h post-glucose*) is conducted after an overnight fast (10–16 h during which only water is consumed). The patient takes 75 g of anhydrous glucose in 250–350 mL of water by mouth. A sample of blood is taken 2 h later for the measurement of venous plasma glucose concentration. A venous plasma glucose value of ≥11.1 mmol/L (140–200 mg/dL) is indicative of impaired glucose tolerance (IGT).

category for subsequent development of diabetes mellitus. People with IFG should have an OGTT to exclude a diagnosis of diabetes.

WHO classification criteria

The revised WHO classification criteria encompasses both the clinical stages and aetiological types of diabetes mellitus and other categories of hyperglycaemia. The clinical staging reflects that diabetes – regardless of its aetiology – progresses through several clinical stages during its natural history. Clinical stages include normoglycaemia, impaired glucose regulation and diabetes mellitus.[4] The classification by aetiological type designates defects, disorders or processes that often result in diabetes mellitus. Aetiological types include type 1 diabetes (formally referred to as insulin-dependent diabetes mellitus), type 2 diabetes (formally referred to as non-insulin-dependent diabetes mellitus) and other specific types.

Type 1 diabetes mellitus

This is characterised by insulin deficiency resulting from immune-mediated pancreatic beta-cell destruction. Type 1 diabetes results from destruction of pancreatic beta-cells, through an autoimmune process of unknown aetiology, leading to insulin deficiency and associated keto-acidosis. Several immunological markers, reflecting ongoing immune activity and possible beta-cell damage, have been identified. These include islet-cell cytoplasmic antibodies (ICA), insulin autoantibodies (IAA) and antibodies to glutamate decarboxylase (anti-GAD). Individuals with no evidence of autoimmunity can be classified as having type 1 idiopathic diabetes. This category does not include forms of diabetes where beta-cell destruction is known to be due to non-immune specific causes, e.g. cystic fibrosis.

Pancreatic beta-cell destruction eventually results in absolute insulin deficiency. The pathological process occurs in genetically predisposed individuals over many years and appears to be triggered by environmental factors such as viral infections and nutritional factors such as ingestion of cow's milk in early childhood. Cow's milk proteins have been found to act as antibodies to the pancreatic beta-cell surface protein. These proteins are identical to the antibodies initially identified as being directed against a sequence of 17 amino acids in bovine serum albumin. Susceptibility to type 1 diabetes may be increased if cow's milk proteins have been consumed during the neonatal period or in early infancy. The immune mechanisms involved during initial stages of the attack on the beta-cells remain to be established. Once the process has been initiated, the beta-cell destruction appears to occur via several different processes including antigen-specific pathways (T-cell-mediated) and non-specific inflammatory responses (cytokine-induced release of free oxygen and nitric acid radicals which in turn damage beta-cells).

Genetic factors

There is an increased risk of developing type 1 diabetes in first-degree relatives, and the incidence is higher in monozygotic twins (25–30%) than in dizygotic twins (5–10%). Genes implicated include the HLA region located on the short arm of chromosome 6, specifically those which regulate the immune response. There is a strong association between type 1 diabetes and some HLA-DQ-encoded heterodimers. In those of European origin, predisposition to type 1 diabetes is associated with HLA-DR3, DQw2 (also known as DQB1*0201) and with HLA-DR4, DQw8 (also known as DQB1*0302). However, there is no single HLA allele or a combination that has been identified as specific for type 1 diabetes, and not all individuals with a particular genetic make-up develop the disease.

The rate of beta-cell destruction is variable. The severity of symptoms on presentation can range from fasting hyperglycaemia in adults with sufficient residual beta-cell function to prevent ketoacidosis for many years to ketoacidosis on presentation in children and adolescents. Type 1 diabetes can also occur in the elderly. Although weight loss is a common symptom of diabetes, some patients may still be obese on presentation.

Individuals with type 1 diabetes become dependent on exogenous insulin for survival and are at risk from ketoacidosis (see pp. 33–34).

Type 2 diabetes mellitus

This is generally characterised by peripheral insulin resistance and relative insulin deficiency which may range from predominant insulin resistance with relative insulin deficiency to predominant insulin secretory defect with insulin resistance. Some patients develop severe insulin deficiency.[3] Obesity is common in people with type 2 diabetes and itself causes insulin resistance. Body fat distribution (see Risk Factors Focus, p. 27) rather than obesity (classified according to body mass index, BMI) may have greater significance in this type of diabetes as many people have increased distribution of fat in the abdominal region (central obesity). Peripheral plasma insulin levels are usually high, with relative insulin deficiency being characterised by a delayed initial first-phase insulin response with the second-phase insulin response being weakened over several years. Resistance to the action of insulin takes the form of a decrease in the ability of skeletal muscle both to store glucose (due to a reduction in activity of the enzyme glycogen synthase) and to oxidise glucose (due to a reduction in pyruvate dehydrogenase activity). There is also an increase in hepatic glucose output (HGO) due to inhibition of glycolysis and an increase in glucogenesis leading to chronic hyperglycaemia. Development of hyperglycaemia is a gradual process which frequently goes undiagnosed for many years due to an absence of any classic symptoms of diabetes during the early stages of the disease.

The risk of developing type 2 diabetes increases with age, obesity (particularly central obesity), family history of diabetes or cardiovascular disease (particularly hypertension or dyslipidaemia), and lack of physical activity. The risk of developing type 2 diabetes is higher, and the average age of diagnosis is younger in people of South Asian, African and African-Caribbean descent and less affluent populations. Compared with the white population, type 2 diabetes is up to six times more common in people of South Asian descent and up to three times more common in people of African and African-Caribbean descent. In these groups the risk of diabetes-related death is between three and six times higher, and these groups are also particularly susceptible to cardiovascular and renal complications of diabetes. The association with a strong genetic predisposition is higher than for type 1 diabetes, but the genetics have not been defined.

Individuals with type 2 diabetes do not require exogenous insulin for survival, although it may be a requirement for glycaemic control in some patients. Non-ketotic hyperosmolar coma may occur as a result of stress from an illness such as infection, particularly in the elderly (see pp. 34–35).

Other specific types

This group categorises diabetes according to specific causes and includes genetic defects in beta-cell function, genetic defects in insulin action, diseases of the exocrine pancreas, endocrinopathies, drug- or chemical-induced, infections, uncommon forms of immune-mediated diabetes, other genetic syndromes sometimes associated with diabetes and gestational diabetes mellitus (GDM).[4]

References

1. Hillson R. *Practical Diabetes Care*. Oxford: Oxford University Press, 1996.
2. Nattrass M (ed.). *Malin's Clinical Diabetes*, 2nd edn. London: Chapman & Hall, 1996.
3. MeReC Bulletin. Non-insulin-dependent diabetes mellitus (part 1). *MeReC Bull* 1996; 7: 21–24.
4. World Health Organization. *Definition, Diagnosis and Classification of Diabetes Mellitus and its complications (Part 1)*. Geneva: World Health Organization, Department of Non-communicable Disease Surveillance, 1999.
5. Department of Health. National Service Framework for Diabetes: Standards 2002. www.doh.gov.uk/nsf/diabetes
6. Scottish Intercollegiate Guidelines Network. *55: Management of Diabetes Quick reference Guide*. November 2001.

3

Prevention and management of diabetic complications

Untreated or poorly controlled diabetes leads to the development of diabetic complications. The onset of type 1 diabetes is fairly rapid; therefore, the majority of type 1 diabetic patients do not have diabetic complications at the time of diagnosis. Many people with type 2 diabetes are not aware that they have diabetes. The disease is present on average for 5–7 years before diagnosis, and approximately 50% of newly diagnosed patients have one or more complications at the time of diagnosis. Diabetic complications can have serious consequences on the health and life of the patient. The risks of the disease can be minimised if good metabolic control can be achieved by using a combination of drug therapy and lifestyle changes. Metabolic targets represent a practical tool with which to monitor disease management. Targets for reducing risk factors can be modified to suit individual patients according to age and the expected degree of compliance.[1]

There are two main categories of diabetic complications:

1. Microvascular complications which are specific to diabetes mellitus.
2. Macrovascular complications which are non-specific.

Microvascular complications

Diabetes mellitus affects the small blood vessels throughout the body. Damage to these blood vessels and the basement membrane impairs the delivery of nutrients and hormones to the tissues, which in turn causes tissue damage. The mechanisms involved in the development of chronic microvascular complications are diverse and remain to be established. Hyperglycaemia inhibits glucose transport (see pp. 82), possibly by down-regulation of GLUT 4 transporters, and chronic hyperglycaemia impairs muscle glucose uptake. Several mechanisms, including direct glucose toxicity, accumulation of advanced glycation end-products (AGEs) and breakdown of glucose to sorbitol via the polyol pathway, are under investigation. The main sites to be affected are the retina, the renal glomerulus and the nerve sheath. Diabetic complications such as retinopathy, nephropathy and peripheral neuropathy can lead to blindness, renal failure and limb amputation, respectively.

Glycaemic control

The Diabetes Control and Complications Trial (DCCT)[2,3] has demonstrated the association between the degree of glycaemic control and the development of microvascular complications in type 1 diabetic patients. Intensive management (i.e. attempting to maintain normoglycaemia) in type 1 diabetic patients decreases the risk (by 40–75%) of development and progression of complications, particularly retinopathy. The risk of hypoglycaemia is increased with intensive management. Epidemiological studies have indicated that the association between glycaemic control and microvascular complications also exists in type 2 diabetes.[4,5] This has now been confirmed by the results of the United Kingdom Prospective Diabetes Study (UKPDS) which was initiated in 1977 to determine whether aiming treatment to achieve normal blood glucose levels (<6.0 mmol/L) prevents the onset of microvascular and macrovascular diabetic complications in diabetic patients. UKPDS 33[6] has demonstrated that intensive management (with sulphonylurea or insulin) of blood glucose levels (11% reduction in median HbA_{1c} over the first 10 years after diagnosis) substantially decreased the risk (by 25%) of microvascular endpoints, particularly in the number of patients requiring photocoagulation therapy. The evidence for reduction in risk of endpoints from macrovascular complications such as myocardial infarction (16% reduction in risk) was inconclusive, and no difference in either diabetes-related mortality or all-cause mortality was found between the intensively managed group and the conventionally managed group. Intensive blood glucose management with either a sulphonylurea or insulin increases the risk of hypoglycaemia. Evidence from UKPDS 34[7] suggests that intensive blood glucose management with metformin decreases the risk of microvascular complications in overweight (>120% ideal bodyweight) diabetic patients. There was no increase in the risk of hypoglycaemia with intensive metformin therapy. For a discussion on individual antidiabetic drugs, see Chapter 7. The blood glucose level regarded as being diagnostic of diabetes is based on the risk of developing the microvascular complications of diabetes: the risk of retinopathy, neuropathy and nephropathy rises abruptly at or around a fasting blood glucose level of 7.0 mmol/L. The higher the blood glucose level, the greater the risk of a person with diabetes developing these long-term complications.[8,9]

Retinopathy

Retinopathy results from damage to the capillaries supplying the retina and is a major cause of blindness in people with diabetes. The risk of developing retinopathy increases with the duration of diabetes and poor blood glucose control. Other risk factors for retinopathy include - hypertension, dyslipidaemia and pregnancy. The onset and progression of diabetic retinopathy can be delayed by intensive blood glucose control and tight control of raised blood pressure.[8] Vision is not affected by all retinopathies; however, prompt treatment is important for controlling the condition and maintaining vision.[10] Micro-angiopathy affecting the retina develops over a number of years. The main types of retinopathy associated with visual loss are proliferative retinopathy (where new blood vessels develop which may lead to haemorrhage and scarring) and maculopathy (where there is capillary blood vessel leakage into the retina). If untreated, 6–9% of people with proliferative retinopathy become blind each year, and 10% of people with macu-lopathy develop moderate visual loss each year. Primary screening is usually performed by optometrists. Secondary screening – that is, in people requiring management decisions – is usually carried out by ophthalmologists. All people with diabetes should receive ophthalmo-logical examinations at least annually.[11] Cataracts and chronic glau-coma are also more common in people with diabetes.[12] Cataracts occur about 10 years earlier in people with diabetes compared to people without diabetes.[8]

Nephropathy

Diabetic nephropathy is caused by damage to the kidney, which results in proteinuria and hypertension, and subsequently a decline in glomeru-lar filtration rate (GFR). Diabetic nephropathy is defined as the presence of clinical proteinuria (urine dipstick persistently positive for protein or albumin excretion >300 mg/day) in a person with diabetes who does not have any other renal disease (see also Risk Factors Focus, p. 14). Nephropathy is a major cause of mortality in diabetic patients. Mortal-ity rates from cardiovascular disease in people with diabetes who also had nephropathy are up to eight times higher than in people who do not

RISK FACTORS FOCUS

Renal function[13]

Normal range

Albumin: creatinine ratio: 2.5 mmol (men); 3.5 mmol (women)
Albumin concentration: <20 mg/L

Microalbuminuria*

Albumin: creatinine ratio ≥2.5 mg/mmol (men); ≥3.5 mg/mmol (women)
Albumin concentration: ≥20 mg/L

Proteinuria

Albumin: creatinine ratio: >30 mg/mmol
Albumin concentration: >200 mg/L

* A transient increase in urinary albumin excretion can be caused by urinary tract infections, cardiac failure, acute illness or heavy exercise.

have diabetic nephropathy. The risk of developing diabetic nephropathy increases with duration of diabetes, level of blood glucose control and age. Other risk factors for the development of nephropathy include raised blood pressure, smoking and dyslipidaemia. Nephropathy is more likely to be present if retinopathy has already been diagnosed. Around 30% of patients with type 1 diabetes develop nephropathy.[16] The incidence in type 2 diabetic patients varies with ethnic origin and ranges from 25% (Europeans) to 50% (African-Caribbean, South Asian and Japanese). The higher incidence in African-Caribbean and South Asians may be due to a higher frequency of arterial hypertension and a younger age of onset on type 2 diabetes, respectively.[13] In people with diabetes who already have nephropathy, tight blood glucose control and tight control of high blood pressure can significantly reduce the rate of progression of nephropathy. Protein restriction can also reduce the decline in renal function.[16]

Stages of diabetic nephropathy[13]

The clinical symptoms of diabetic nephropathy develop over several years. Early changes in renal function include glomerular hyperfiltration, increased renal blood flow and hypertrophy of the kidney.

Micro-albuminuria (incipient nephropathy)   Micro-albuminuria (albumin excretion rate 20–200 mg/min or 30–300 mg/day for at least two out of three consecutive sterile urine specimens) is the first sign of diabetic nephropathy.

Management should focus on:

- Glycaemic control. The DCCT and UKPDS trials have demonstrated that the better the glycaemic control, the lower the risk of developing micro-albuminuria. Suggested upper limits for HbA_{1c} (DCCT-aligned) are 7.5% for those on insulin and 7.0% for others. There is little evidence that improving glycaemic control changes progression to nephropathy.
- Blood pressure control. Increased arterial pressure can cause damage to the kidneys. In type 2 diabetes, the lower the blood pressure, the lower the risk of developing microalbuminuria. Suggested upper limits are 140/80 mmHg (see Risk Factors Focus, p. 21).
- Blood lipids. Elevated levels of cholesterol and triglycerides (see Risk Factors Focus, p. 22) may be associated with micro-albuminuria. Weight reduction and dietary restriction should be considered. Long-term data on effect of lipid-lowering interventions are lacking.
- Smoking. This should be discouraged as it is associated with the development of micro-albuminuria.

Macro-albuminuria (clinical nephropathy)   Patients with macro-albuminuria have an albumin excretion rate of >200 mg/min or >300 mg/day. Diabetic retinopathy is usually present (its absence may indicate a non-diabetic cause of proteinuria). Arterial hypertension with hypo-albuminaemia, peripheral oedema, lipid disturbances and athero-sclerotic complications are usually prominent. Strict glycaemic control does not appear to have the effect of slowing down the progression of clinical nephropathy. Oral antidiabetic therapy should be replaced with insulin in people with type 2 diabetes and a GFR of <30 mL/min.

Chlorpropamide, glibenclamide and metformin are not suitable for use in people with type 2 diabetes and impaired renal function.

Management should consider the following:

- Blood pressure control. Drug treatment of hypertension. ACE inhibitors may offer an additional independent benefit (see Management Focus, p. 23). Target blood pressure is <120/70 mmHg for people with type 1 diabetes and <135/75 mmHg for people with type 2 diabetes.
- Protein restriction. A reduction in animal protein intake and replacement of animal with vegetable sources of protein should be considered.

Vegetable protein appears to be less damaging to the kidney. Any restriction in protein intake should be undertaken under supervision in order to avoid problems with low-protein diets.

- Blood lipids. Abnormal lipid profiles may contribute to the progression of renal failure and cardiovascular complications. Data on the effect of lipid-lowering on the progression of renal failure are lacking. Correction of hyperlipidaemia has a beneficial effect on the outcome of cardiovascular disease (see pp. 21–22).
- Smoking. This is associated with poor prognosis.

Uraemia (end-stage renal failure) Uraemia is persistent albuminuria with a gradual decline in the GFR. Management includes renal dialysis or kidney transplantation. High serum urea concentrations may cause carbamylation of haemoglobin and therefore make the measurement of glycated haemoglobin (see p. 52) unreliable. The gross changes in serum albumin concentration need to be taken into consideration if glycaemic control is being monitored by measurement of serum fructosamine (see p. 52). Good glycaemic control is important both before and after kidney transplantation.

Neuropathy

Diabetic neuropathy is usually symmetrical and mainly affects the sensory nervous system. Symptoms include pain (sharp, stabbing or burning, particularly on the shins and soles of feet), skin tenderness and a feeling of numbness.[24] However, approximately 50% of the affected patients may be asymptomatic. The symptoms of autonomic neuropathy include impotence, gastrointestinal dysfunction and lack of sweating in the feet. Symptoms of cardiac autonomic neuropathy include resting tachycardia and a fall in systolic blood pressure on standing. Mononeuropathies are also common in diabetic patients.

Management of symptoms of common diabetic neuropathies[24]

Sensorimotor neuropathy

- Pain. The pain of diabetic neuropathy does not respond to conventional analgesics and it can be extremely distressing. A dramatic relief in symptoms (within 48 h) has been reported with the tricyclic antidepressants imipramine and amitriptyline. Postural hypotension may be a problem in patients with autonomic neuropathy. Carbamazepine and phenytoin have also been used. Capsaicin inhibits neuronal transmission when applied topically as a cream (Axsain, manufactured by Bioglan) and is now available for the treatment of painful diabetic neuropathy. Although it does not provide instant relief, pain relief increases with continued use for more than 4 weeks. The lack of systemic side effects offers an advantage over tricylic antidepressants. Patients should be advised to carefully follow the application instructions for capsaicin cream.[25]

- Skin tenderness. Symptoms may be improved by covering the affected area with a vapour-permeable film dressing such as Tegaderm.[24]

Autonomic neuropathy

- Postural hypotension. A drop in systolic blood pressure of >10 mmHg on standing. Symptoms may be alleviated by the patient sleeping with the head of the bed elevated, by the use of support stockings, or by taking fludrocortisone (caution if oedema occurs or if there is hypertension when the patient is lying down).[24]
- Gustatory sweating. An anticholinergic drug such as propantheline may help relieve abnormal facial sweating while eating.[24]
- Gastroparesis. Metoclopramide, domperidone and cisapride are used to relieve the nausea and vomiting caused by gastroparesis.[24]
- Male impotence. Erectile failure affects up to 30% of men with diabetes. Treatment options are the same as for erectile dysfunction from other causes.[26]

The diabetic foot

Peripheral neuropathy can cause symmetric sensory loss in the feet and legs, resulting in the loss of protective sensation in the feet. The loss of protective sensation in combination with vascular impairment (diminished blood flow) and infection can lead to development of the 'diabetic foot'. Neuronal and vascular complications can cause small lesions or ulcers to develop on the foot from dry skin. These may go unnoticed by the patient (due to impairment in sensory nerve function) until severe infection or gangrene becomes established. Patients with diabetes must be evaluated for risk of developing foot lesions.[27] Diabetic patients with sensory loss or vascular disease possibly with structural, skin or nail deformities are at high risk of developing foot ulcers, and should be seen at frequent intervals by a qualified professional with experience in the care of diabetic foot problems. These patients need to be educated on the role of the loss of sensory protection in foot injury and taught how to perform daily foot care. They should avoid repetitive weight-bearing exercise such as jogging, step exercises and prolonged walking. Diabetic patients who are not at high risk should be educated to understand basic preventative measures for foot care and have their feet inspected routinely. Basic preventative measures include foot hygiene, well-fitted footwear, daily inspection of feet, avoidance of foot trauma (e.g. by not going about barefoot), and seeking professional help if problems occur, i.e. avoiding self-care of ingrown toenails, corns or athlete's foot.[28] All those who develop new swelling, redness, discoloration, pain or ulceration of their feet should be referred urgently (usually within 24 h) to a multidisciplinary foot care service.[29]

Macrovascular complications

Type 2 diabetes usually presents as a syndrome of metabolic abnormalities which include hyperglycaemia, central obesity, dyslipidaemia, hypercoagulation, hypertension and insulin resistance. Large-vessel disease, including deposition of large fatty plaques in arteries, increases the risk of stroke and myocardial infarction. The most common cause of mortality and morbidity in people with diabetes, particularly type 2 diabetes, is coronary heart disease. The risk of developing coronary heart disease is higher in people with diabetes (two to three times higher in men and four to five times higher in premenopausal women), and the prevalence of coronary heart disease is higher in people of South Asian descent with diabetes compared with Europeans with diabetes. The risk of ischaemic heart disease is twice as high in South Asians compared with Europeans with diabetes. Stroke is also more common in people with diabetes, particularly in people of African and African-Caribbean descent.[8] However, one study has shown that different sub-groups of people of South Asian descent such as Indians, Pakistanis and Bangladeshis differ in a wide range of coronary risk factors and combining their data is misleading.[30] Five, potentially modifiable, risk factors for coronary artery disease in European people with type 2 diabetes have been identified[14]; these include hyperglycaemia, hypertension, increased low-density lipoprotein (LDL)-cholesterol, decreased high-density lipoprotein (HDL)-cholesterol and smoking (see Risk Factors Focus, p. 19).

The study UKPDS 23[14] has found that obesity (including central obesity), raised insulin concentrations and decreased physical activity were not major risk factors for coronary artery disease in type 2 diabetes, although these factors provide an increased risk for cardiovascular

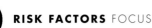

RISK FACTORS FOCUS

Potentially modifiable risk factors for coronary artery disease in white diabetic patients[14]

- Increased concentration of low-density lipoprotein (LDL) -cholesterol. An increment of 1.0 mmol/L ≡ 1.57-fold increase in risk
- Decreased concentration of high-density lipoprotein (HDL) -cholesterol. An increment of 0.1 mmol/L ≡ 0.15-fold decrease in risk
- Raised blood pressure. An increment of 10 mmHg systolic blood pressure ≡ 1.15-fold increase in risk
- Hyperglycaemia (measured as HbA_{1c}). An increment of 1% ≡ 1.11-fold increase in risk
- Smoking

---

disease in the general population. The study indicates that although these variables are risk factors for the development of diabetes mellitus, once the diabetes has developed, the five risk factors (increased LDL-cholesterol, decreased HDL-cholesterol, hypertension, hyperglycaemia and smoking) represent a greater risk for coronary artery disease. Whether modification of these risk factors reduces the prevalence of coronary artery disease in patients with type 2 diabetes mellitus remains to be established. The recommendations for reducing the risk of coronary events are set out in terms of 'higher' and 'lower' 10-year coronary event risk (see Risk Factors Focus, p. 20).[15]

Hypertension

Hypertension is an independent risk factor for cardiovascular, cerebral, renal and peripheral atherosclerotic vascular disease. Its prevalence in diabetic patients is approximately twice that in the non-diabetic population, and is more common in men with diabetes under the age of 50 years and in women with diabetes over the age of 50 years. The prevalence of hypertension increases with age, obesity and the duration of diabetes.

High blood pressure increases the risk of diabetic nephropathy and cardiovascular disease. High systolic blood pressure (≥160 mmHg) is a strong risk factor and is associated with a two- to four-fold increase in the mortality of diabetic patients. The severity of retinopathy has also been associated with hypertension.[23] An evaluation (UKPDS 38) of whether intensive management of hypertension prevents macrovascular and microvascular complications in type 2 diabetic patients has

RISK FACTORS FOCUS

Assessing the 10-year coronary event risk[15]

The 10-year coronary event risk is defined as 'higher risk' and 'lower risk' in the national clinical guidelines.

Higher risk

- presence of cardiovascular disease (a history of symptoms of coronary heart disease, stroke or peripheral vascular disease); *or*
- a 10-year coronary event risk assessed as >15% according to Coronary Risk Prediction Charts*

Lower risk

- no cardiovascular disease; *and*
- a 10-year coronary event risk ≤15% according to Coronary Risk Prediction Charts*

---

* Joint British Societies Coronary Risk Prediction Chart. *Heart* 1998; 80: S1–S29. Also reproduced in the *British National Formulary*

---

demonstrated that tight control of blood pressure (mean 144/82 mmHg over 9 years) significantly reduces the risk of microvascular complications (37%), stroke (44%), heart failure (56%) and death related to diabetes (32%). There is also a significant reduction in risk (24%) for any endpoint related to diabetes.[17]

Type 1 diabetes

Blood pressure usually remains within the normal range for the first 5–10 years of diabetes. Hypertension, characterised by the elevation of both systolic and diastolic blood pressure, typically develops with the onset of renal disease. Long-term (>30 years) survivors of diabetes who have not developed diabetic nephropathy rarely have hypertension.

Type 2 diabetes

Patients frequently have hypertension at the time of diagnosis of diabetes. It has been suggested that hormonal or metabolic abnormalities associated with hypertension may exacerbate glucose intolerance, or that both conditions have a common underlying mechanism. Hypertension and type 2 diabetes share certain risk factors such as obesity, visceral adiposity and possibly insulin resistance. Insulin resistance and hyperinsulinaemia have been proposed as a link between hypertension and glucose intolerance but the underlying mechanism remains unclear. The contribution of impaired renal function to the development of hypertension is not well defined. Isolated systolic hypertension is common in type 2 diabetes and has been attributed to macrovascular disease and the loss of elastic compliance in large arteries.

Non-drug treatment of hypertension includes weight reduction, regular exercise (see p. 39), and reductions in both salt (see p. 62) and alcohol intakes. Determining factors for the choice of antihypertensive drug therapy include age, ethnic origin, gender and other concurrent conditions such as renal, cardiovascular or peripheral vascular disease (see Management Focus, pp. 23–25).[18] A comparison of the effects of captopril (ACE inhibitor) and atenolol (cardioselective beta-blocker) in reducing the incidence of diabetic complications has shown no difference between the two types of drug therapy, and the study UKPDS 39 suggests that the important factor is the reduction in blood pressure itself rather than the therapy used.[19]

Dyslipidaemias

Lipid and lipoprotein abnormalities are common in diabetes, particularly type 2 diabetes.[32] Plasma cholesterol is an independent risk factor for coronary heart disease. The risk is higher in people with diabetes

RISK FACTORS FOCUS

Monitoring blood pressure in people with diabetes[15]	
Blood pressure	Recommendation
<140/80 mmHg	Monitor on an annual basis. If blood pressure is 140/80 mmHg or above, confirm with two further readings over a period of 2 months
≥140/80 mmHg and <160/100 mmHg	If *lower coronary event risk**, monitor every 6 months or more frequently if necessary.
	If *higher coronary event risk** OR concomitant microalbuminuria present regardless of coronary event risk, aim for a target blood pressure <140/80 mmHg with pharmacological treatment to reduce blood pressure

*For definition of coronary event risk, see Risk Factor Focus, p. 20.

than in the non-diabetic population. High levels of LDL-cholesterol or triglycerides increase the risk, whereas high levels of HDL-cholesterol appear to have a protective effect. Total triglyceride levels appear to be related to the risk of coronary heart disease, but the exact nature of the relationship is unclear.[33] Determination of the lipid profile (total cholesterol, fasting triglyceride and HDL-cholesterol) should form a part of the annual assessment of the diabetic patient (see Risk Factors Focus, below).

Type 1 diabetes

In patients with good glycaemic control, plasma lipid and lipoprotein concentrations are usually within the range for the non-diabetic population. Increased cholesterol, LDL-cholesterol and triglycerides and decreased HDL-cholesterol are associated with the onset of diabetic

RISK FACTORS FOCUS

Monitoring blood lipids profile in type 2 diabetes[17]	
Blood lipids profile	*Recommendation*
TC <5.0 mmol/L *or* LDL-C <3.0 mmol/L *and* TG <2.3 mmol/L	Monitor annually
TC >5.0 mmol/L *or* LDL-C ≥3.0 mmol/L *or* TG ≥2.3 mmol/L but <10 mmol/L	Check alcohol consumption, thyroid function, hepatic and renal function. Offer advice on diet and physical activity. If *lower coronary event risk**, consider statin therapy at higher levels of TC or TG If *higher coronary event risk**, statin therapy
TC <5.0 mmol/L *or* LDL-C <3.0 mmol/L *and* TG ≥2.3 mmol/L but <10 mmol/L	If *higher coronary event risk**, statin or fibrate therapy
Fasting TG ≥10 mmol/L	Regardless of *coronary event risk**, specialist management required

TC: total cholesterol; LDL-C: low-density lipoproteins; TG: triglycerides.
* For definition of coronary event risk, see Risk Factor Focus, p. 20.

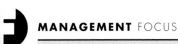

MANAGEMENT FOCUS

Antihypertensive drug therapy in diabetic patients[18]

Angiotensin-converting enzyme (ACE) inhibitors *Captopril, Cilazapril, Enalapril Fosinopril, Lisinopril, Moexipril, Perindopril, Quinapril, Ramipril, Trandolapril*	Used as first-line therapy in patients with microalbuminuria, proteinuria or nephropathy, as the effect of delaying the progression of diabetic renal disease is independent of the antihypertensive effect; however, no evidence for this renal protective was found in UKPDS 39.[19] ACE inhibitors are also useful for the management of heart failure in diabetic patients.[20] A potentially serious interaction between ACE inhibitors and aspirin has been reported; see under Aspirin, below. ACE inhibitors may enhance the hypoglycaemic effect of antidiabetic drugs (see p. 94). ACE inhibitors are less effective in patients of African-Caribbean origin and in the elderly. ACE inhibitors should be used with caution in advanced renal disease and possible renal stenosis
Calcium channel blockers (calcium channel antagonists) *Amlodipine, Diltiazem, Felodipine, Isradipine, Lacidipine, Mibefradil, Nicardipine, Nisoldipine, Verapamil*	Usually well tolerated. Also have anti-anginal effects. African-Caribbeans are more sensitive to calcium channel blocker therapy. Calcium channel blockers may affect glucose tolerance (see Management Focus, p. 29). Peripheral oedema may be a problem with some calcium channel blockers in the presence of peripheral sensory neuropathy. Avoid in heart failure. The suggestion that calcium channel blockers may increase the risk of myocardial infarction in diabetic patients is controversial.[21] A possible explanation is that the higher rate of coronary events noted

continued overleaf

Management Focus (continued)

in hypertensive diabetic patients with ACE inhibitors is due to the protective effect of ACE inhibitors rather than damage caused by calcium channel blockers[22]

Diuretics
Loop: *Frusemide, Bumetanide, Torasemide, Ethacrynic acid*
Potassium-sparing: *Amiloride, Triamterene, Spironolactone*
Thiazide: *Bendrofluazide, Chlorothiazide, Chlorthalidone Cyclopenthiazide, Hydrochlorothiazide, Hydroflumethiazide, Indapamide, Merfruside, Metolazone, Polythiazide, Xipamide*

Thiazide diuretics in small doses are effective in lowering blood pressure. They have been reported to cause short-term dyslipidaemia, altered carbohydrate metabolism, hyperinsulinaemia, hypokalaemia, hypomagnesaemia and hyperuricaemia in some patients (see also Management Focus, p. 29).[23] *Loop diuretics* may affect glucose tolerance (see Management Focus, p. 29). *Potassium-sparing diuretics* increase the risk of hyperkalaemia in diabetic patients. Patients of African-Caribbean origin are more sensitive to diuretic therapy

Beta-blockers
(Beta-adrenoceptor blocking drugs)
Acebutolol, Atenolol, Betaxolol, Bisoprolol, Carvedilol, Celiprolol, Esmolol, Labetalol, Metoprolol, Nadolol, Oxprenolol, Pindolol, Propranolol

Cardioselective beta-blockers are preferred. Non-selective beta-blockers can have adverse effects on glycaemic control and lipid levels and can also reduce hypoglycaemic awareness (see Management Focus, p. 29 and also pp. 94–96).[23] Patients of African-Caribbean origin are less sensitive to beta-blocker therapy

Alpha-blockers
Doxazosin, Indoramin, Prazosin, Terazosin

May improve insulin sensitivity and have a beneficial effect on lipoproteins (reduced low-density lipoproteins and increased high-density lipoproteins). Orthostatic hypotension may be a problem in diabetic patients with autonomic neuropathy

continued overleaf

Management Focus (continued)

Angiotensin II antagonists
Candesartan, Irbesartan, Losartan, Valsartan

Data on long-term outcome in diabetic patients not available. Action similar to ACE inhibitors but fewer side effects. May be useful in patients not able to tolerate ACE inhibitors

---

nephropathy. Lipaemia with very high triglyceride levels may develop in diabetic ketoacidosis due to marked insulin deficiency (see p. 33). The atherogenic potential of lipoproteins may be increased by glycation; for example glycation of apoprotein B reduces its affinity for the LDL receptor and makes it available for uptake by macrophage scavenger receptors leading to the formation of foam cells and 'fatty streaks'.

Type 2 diabetes

Lipid and lipoprotein abnormalities are common in patients with type 2 diabetes. Insulin deficiency and insulin resistance are associated with alterations in lipid metabolism. Prolonged post-prandial lipaemia, hypertriglyceridaemia (characterised by the accumulation of atherogenic remnant particles from partial hydrolysis of VLDL) and low HDL-cholesterol are the major abnormalities. There is also an increase in the proportion of small, dense LDL particles which are potentially athero-genic because of their susceptibility to oxidation and greater binding affinity for the arterial wall.

There is strong evidence of the beneficial effect of lipid lowering in both the diabetic and non-diabetic population. Management of dyslipid-aemia in diabetic patients is similar to that for the non-diabetic popu-lation. Initial management involves achieving good glycaemic control (see Glycaemic Control Focus, p. 48), weight reduction, exercise (see p. 39) and dietary changes.[35] Statins (HMG-CoA reductase inhibitors) and fibrates are useful for the management of hyperlipidaemia in dia-betic patients (see Management Focus, p. 26). Evidence from the sub-group of diabetic patients (202 out of 4444) with coronary artery disease and hypercholesterolaemia in the Scandinavian Simvastatin Survival Study (4S) indicates that lowering cholesterol with simvastatin reduces the incidence of major coronary events by 55% compared with 32% in the non-diabetic population. The Cholesterol and Recurrent Events

Lipid-lowering drugs[33]

Drugs	Comments
Statins (HMG-CoA reductase inhibitors) *Atrovastatin, Cerivastatin, Fluvastatin, Pravastatin, Simvastatin*	Limit cholesterol synthesis by inhibition of the enzyme HMG-CoA reductase. Useful if hypercholesterolaemia is the major abnormality. Increased risk of myopathy if used in combination with fibrates
Fibrates *Enzafibrate, Ciprofibrate, Clofibrate, Fenofibrate, Gemfibrozil*	Lower triglycerides and increased HDL possibly through stimulation of the peroxisome proliferation system. Some fibrates also reduce fibrinogen concentrations. Useful for hypertriglyceridaemia and low HDL-cholesterol. Increased risk of myopathy if used in combination with statins. Hypoglycaemic effect of sulphonylureas may be enhanced (see p. 110)
Anion-exchange resins *Cholestyramine, Colestipol*	Lower LDL-cholesterol by preventing intestinal reabsorption of bile acids. Hypertriglyceridaemia can be exacerbated. Occasionally used for isolated hypercholesterolaemia in patients who do not want to take systemically acting drugs. Effect of acarbose may be enhanced (see p. 121) and absorption of glipizide reduced (see p. 111) by cholestyramine
Nicotinic acid (and nicotinic acid analogue acipimox)	Inhibits hepatic output of VLDL. Exacerbates hyperglycaemia, therefore not used in diabetic patients
Fish oil supplements (w-3 Marine triglycerides – *Maxepa*)	Possibly reduce hepatic output of VLDL May aggravate hypercholesterolaemia and exacerbate hyperglycaemia

(CARE) trial found no distinction in the reduction in coronary events with pravastatin treatment between the diabetic (25% reduction) and non-diabetic populations (23% reduction).[36,37]

There is evidence that lowering cholesterol is beneficial in people with diabetes but with no evidence of cardiovascular disease and either 'normal' or borderline raised cholesterol. The Heart Protection Study evaluated over 20 000 people aged between 40 and 80 years and included about 4000 people with diabetes, cholesterol within normal or low range, and no history of coronary heart disease. The key finding of the study was that coronary heart disease events were reduced by 25% in people receiving simvastatin 40 mg daily. This beneficial effect appeared to be independent of age or the total cholesterol levels at entry into the trial.[38]

Obesity

Obesity (in the UK defined as body mass index >30; see Risk Factors Focus, below) is highly prevalent among hypertensive and type 2 diabetic patients. Obesity increases insulin resistance and is a risk factor for the development of type 2 diabetes (see pp. 8–9).[34] It is a major risk factor for cardiovascular disease in the general population, but not for coronary artery disease in diabetic patients (see Risk Factors Focus, p. 19).[12,34] Weight reduction can lead to an improvement in insulin sensitivity, reduce blood pressure and improve the blood lipids profile.[39]

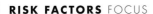

RISK FACTORS FOCUS

Body mass index. Body weight (kg)/height (m)^2.[12]			
	Good	Acceptable	Poor
Men	<25	25–27	>27
Women	<24	24–26	>26

The body mass index (BMI) is a crude measurement of obesity as it does not differentiate the different components of body weight, i.e. the proportion of weight due to fat, bone and muscle. The recommended ideal body mass index for adults is 20–27 kg/m^2. Other units of measurement of obesity include the waist:hip ratio (WHR), which is considered to reflect the pattern of body fat distribution and hence have a greater relevance to cardiovascular disease. Men who have a WHR >0.95 and women who have a WHR >0.85 are considered to have central obesity. Obesity has also been defined in terms of the waist circumference. Risk of type 2 diabetes and cardiovascular disease is considered to be significantly increased if the waist circumference is >80 cm in women and >94 cm in men.[34]

Antiplatelet therapy

Platelets make a major contribution to atherosclerosis and vascular disease. Platelets from diabetic subjects have been found to be hypersensitive to platelet aggregating agents *in vitro*. A possible mechanism is an increase in the production of thromboxane (potent vasoconstrictor and platelet-aggregating agent), evidence for which has been found in type 2 diabetic patients with cardiovascular disease.

Aspirin

Aspirin blocks thromboxane synthesis and has been used in the prevention of cardiovascular events for both diabetic and non-diabetic subjects. Evidence suggests that low-dose aspirin (75 mg, enteric-coated preparation) can be used as part of a secondary prevention strategy after cardiovascular events (e.g. after myocardial infarction or transient ischaemic attack) if no contraindications (allergy, bleeding tendency, anticoagulant therapy, gastrointestinal bleeding or clinically active hepatic disease) exist. It may also be used as part of a primary prevention strategy in diabetic patients who are at high risk of cardiovascular events, for example with a family history of coronary disease, smoking, hypertension, obesity, albuminuria, or adverse lipid profile.[40,41] Small doses of aspirin (75 mg daily) used in conjunction with antihypertensive therapy reduces the risk of myocardial infarction in hypertensive patients without increasing the incidence of cerebral bleeding, but with double the incidence of non-fatal major bleeds (e.g. nose bleeds).[15,22]

Interaction with ACE inhibitors

ACE inhibitor therapy in patients with heart failure reduces mortality, but the addition of aspirin therapy does not improve the prognosis in these patients. One of the possible explanations put forward is that aspirin may be negating the benefits of ACE inhibitor therapy. This effect may possibly be due to a different response in heart failure patients to inhibitors of prostaglandin synthesis, retention of sodium due to aspirin or enhanced prostaglandin synthesis due to ACE inhibitors. However, firm evidence of a harmful interaction between ACE inhibitors and aspirin is lacking.[42]

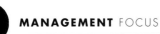

MANAGEMENT FOCUS

Drugs impairing glucose tolerance[43]

Beta$_2$-agonists: The adrenergic system plays a counter-regulatory role to insulin in maintaining glucose homeostasis.

Beta-blockers: Non-selective beta-blockers block pancreatic beta$_2$ receptors associated with insulin release and may inhibit sulphonylurea-induced insulin release in diabetic patients. The clinical relevance of the interaction between sulphonylureas and beta blockers has not been established. For a discussion on the effect of beta blockers on hypoglycaemic awareness, see pp. 94–96.

Calcium channel blockers: Insulin secretion and glucose utilisation are affected by calcium channel blockers. Isolated reports of disturbance of diabetic control with diltiazem, nicardipine and nifedipine.

Chlorpromazine: High doses of chlorpromazine (>100 mg daily) increase blood glucose levels either by inhibiting insulin release or by stimulating the release of adrenaline. This effect is not apparent with lower doses (50–70 mg daily), and clinical evidence of a similar effect with other phenothiazines is lacking. It may be necessary to increase the dose of the hypoglycaemic drug if high-dose chlorpromazine is used concomitantly.

Corticosteroids: The effects of insulin are antagonised by corticosteroids and therefore they have an 'intrinsic hyperglycaemic activity'. Closely monitor diabetic control if corticosteroids are used in a diabetic patient.

Diuretics: Altered carbohydrate metabolism and hyperglycaemia have been reported with thiazide and loop diuretics during long-term use. The hyperglycaemic effect of diuretics may be due to inhibition of insulin secretion and reduced tissue sensitivity to insulin. These effects may partially be related to diuretic-induced hypokalaemia. Increases in blood glucose levels have been reported with frusemide, but diabetic control is not usually affected.

Oral contraceptives: Ethinyloestradiol and progestogens (with high androgenic activity) can cause adverse effects on glycaemic control and lipids profile at high doses. Low-dose contraceptives do not have a significant effect on diabetic control, but monitoring is advisable as some women may require an adjustment in dosage of their antidiabetic therapy.

Phenytoin: Impairs insulin release and may cause hyperglycaemia on long-term therapy. There is a lack of information on the effect of long-term, concomitant use of phenytoin with sulphonylureas.

MANAGEMENT FOCUS

Summary of the aims and components of diabetes management

Aims

- Good blood glucose (glycaemic) control
- Good control of blood pressure
- Attention to plasma lipids
- No smoking

Components

- Diabetes education for patients and their carers
- Dietary control (see Chapter 6)
- Pharmacotherapeutic intervention with antidiabetic drugs (see Chapter 7)
- Monitoring for glycaemic control (see Chapter 5)
- Monitoring for and management of diabetic complications

References

1. Department of Health. National Service Framework for Diabetes: Standards 2002. Interventions. www.doh.gov.uk/nsf/diabetes

2. The Diabetes Control and Complications Trial Research Group. The effect of intensive treatment of diabetes on the development and progression of long-term complications in insulin-dependent diabetes mellitus. *N Engl J Med* 1993; 329: 977–986.

3. British Diabetic Association. Implementing the lessons of DCCT. Report of the national workshop under the auspices of the British Diabetic Association. *Diabetes Med* 1994; 11: 220–228.

4. Nathan D M. Inferences and implications. Do results from the Diabetes Control and Complications Trial apply in NIDDM? *Diabetes Care* 1995; 18: 251–257.

5. Zimmerman B R. Glycaemia control in diabetes mellitus. Towards the normal profile? *Drugs* 1994; 47: 611–621.

6. UK Prospective Diabetes Study (UKPDS) Group. Intensive blood-glucose control with sulphonylureas or insulin compared with conventional treatment and risk of complications in patients with type 2 diabetes (UKPDS 33). *Lancet* 1998; 352: 837–853.

7. UK Prospective Diabetes Study (UKPDS) Group. Effect of intensive blood-glucose control with metformin on complications in overweight patients with type 2 diabetes (UKPDS 34). *Lancet* 1998; 352: 854–865.

8. Department of Health. National Service Framework for Diabetes: Standards 2002. Supplementary information. www.doh.gov.uk/nsf/diabetes

9. Royal College of General Practitioners Effective Clinical Practice Unit. Clinical Guidelines for Type 2 Diabetes: Management of Blood Glucose, 2002. www.nice.org.uk

10. Shilling J. Diabetic retinopathy. *Medicine* 1997; 25: 42–45.

11. Royal College of General Practitioners Effective Clinical Practice Unit. Clinical Guidelines for Type 2 Diabetes: Diabetic Retinopathy: early management and screening, 2002. www.nice.org.uk

12. British Diabetic Association. *Recommendations for the Management of Diabetes in Primary Care*. Diabetes Services Advisory Committee, British Diabetic Association, 1993.

13. Viberti G. Diabetic nephropathy. *Medicine* 1997; 25: 32–35.

14. Turner R C, Millns H, Neil H A W, *et al*. Risk factors for coronary artery disease in non-insulin dependent diabetes mellitus: United Kingdom prospective diabetes study (UKPDS 23). *Br Med J* 1998; 316: 823–828.

15. Royal College of General Practitioners Effective Clinical Practice Unit. Clinical Guidelines for Type 2 Diabetes: Blood Pressure Management, 2002. www.nice.org.uk

16. Royal College of General Practitioners Effective Clinical Practice Unit. Clinical Guidelines for Type 2 Diabetes: Diabetic renal disease: prevention and early management, 2002. www.nice.org.uk

17. Royal College of General Practitioners Effective Clinical Practice Unit. Clinical Guidelines for Type 2 Diabetes: Lipids Management, 2002. www.nice.org.uk

18. Macleod K M, Tooke J E. Diabetes: prescribing antihypertensives, HRT and contraceptives. *Medicine* 1997; 25: 59–61.

19. UK Prospective Diabetes Study (UKPDS) Group. Efficacy of atenolol and captopril in reducing risk of macrovascular and microvascular complications in type 2 diabetes (UKPDS 39). *Br Med J* 1998; 317: 713–720.

20. DiGregorio R V. Managing heart failure in diabetic patients. *Pharmacist* June 1998; 101–112.

21. Stanton A V. Calcium channel blockers. The jury is still out on whether they cause heart attacks and suicide. *Br Med J* 1998; 316: 1471–1473.

22. Hansson L, Zanchetti A, Carruthers S G, *et al*. Effects of intensive blood-pressure lowering and low-dose aspirin in patients with hypertension: principal results of the Hypertension Optimal Treatment (HOT) randomised trial. *Lancet* 1998; 351: 1755–1762.

23. American Diabetes Association Consensus Statement. Treatment of hypertension in diabetes. *Diabetes Care* 1993; 16: 1394–1401.

24. Macleod A F. Diabetic neuropathy. *Medicine* 1997; 25: 36–38.

25. Beckwith S. Product focus: Axsain. *Practice Nursing* 1998; 9: 45–46.

26. Alexander W. Male erectile failure (impotence) and diabetes. *Medicine* 1997; 25(7): 46–47.

27. American Diabetes Association Position Statement. Foot care in patients with diabetes mellitus. *Diabetes Care* 1998; 21 (Supplement 1): S54–S55.

28. Knowles E A, Jackson N J. Care of the diabetic foot. An update on the assessment and treatment of foot lesions in people with diabetes. *J Wound Care* 1997; 6: 227–230.

29. Royal College of General Practitioners Effective Clinical Practice Unit. Clinical Guidelines for Type 2 Diabetes: Prevention and Management of Foot Problems, 2000. www.nice.org.uk

30. Bhopal R, Unwin N, White M, *et al*. Heterogeneity of coronary heart disease risk factors in Indian, Pakistani, Bangladeshi, and European origin populations: cross sectional study. *Br Med J* 1999: 319: 215–220.

31. UK Prospective Diabetes Study (UKPDS) Group. Tight blood pressure control and risk of macrovascular and microvascular complications in type 2 diabetes: (UKPDS 38). *Br Med J* 1998; 317: 703–713.

32. American Diabetes Association Position Statement. Management of dyslipidemia in adults with diabetes. *Diabetes Care* 1998; 21 (Supplement 1): S36–S39.

33. Betteridge D J. Lipids in diabetes. *Medicine* 1997; 25: 48–50.

34. Shaper A G, Wannamethee S G, Walker M. Body weight: implications for the prevention of coronary heart disease, stroke, and diabetes mellitus in a cohort study of middle-aged men. *Br Med J* 1997; 314: 1311–1317.

35. American Diabetes Association Consensus Statement. Detection and management of lipid disorders in diabetes. *Diabetes Care* 1993; 16: 828–834.

36. Hsueh W A, Law R E. Cardiovascular risk continuum: implications of insulin resistance and diabetes. *Am J Med* 1998; 105: 4S–14S.

37. The Scandinavian Simvastatin Survival Study (4S) Group. Cholesterol lowering with simvastatin improves prognosis of diabetic patients with coronary heart disease. A subgroup analysis of the Scandinavian Simvastatin Survival Study (4S). *Diabetes Care* 1997; 20: 614–620.

38. Heart Protection Study Collaborative Group. MRC/BHF Heart protection study of cholesterol lowering with simvastatin in 20536 high risk individuals: a randomised placebo-controlled trial. *Lancet* 2002; 360: 7–22.

39. Wilding J. Obesity treatment. *Br Med J* 1997; 315: 997–1000.

40. American Diabetes Association position statement. Aspirin therapy in diabetes. *Diabetes Care* 1998; 21 (Supplement 1): S45–S46.

41. Yudkin J S. Which diabetic patients should be taking aspirin? *Br Med J* 1995; 311: 641–642.

42. Anonymous. Aspirin/ACE inhibitor interaction? *Pharm J* 1995; 255: 491.

43. O'Byrne S, Feely J. Effects of drugs on glucose tolerance in non-insulin-dependent diabetes. *Drugs* 1990; 40: 6–18 (part I), 203–219 (part II).

4

Lifestyle management

Patients usually associate diabetes mellitus with debilitating complications that result in a loss of independence. The maintenance of near-normal blood glucose levels is the key to avoiding both metabolic (diabetic) emergencies and long-term complications in diabetic patients. The motivation of patients to take responsibility for the day-to-day management of their condition is essential. In order to achieve independence, patients require information and education from health professionals on how to detect, manage and avoid common problems (particularly hypoglycaemia and ketoacidosis) associated with diabetes mellitus.

Ketoacidosis

Diabetic ketoacidosis is an acute and potentially life-threatening complication of diabetes that commonly occurs during illness unusually in uncontrolled type 1 diabetes but can also occur in people with type 2 diabetes in response to acute stress. In adults it can occur over one to two days. The clinical symptoms of ketoacidosis include increased thirst, increased urination, tiredness, nausea and vomiting, smell of acetone on the breath, hyperventilation (air hunger), and occasionally abdominal pain. People with diabetes should be advised to test their urine for ketones if their blood glucose is high (>15 mmol/L) or if they have any of the symptoms of ketoacidosis.

In ketoacidosis, insulin deficiency leads to an increase in hepatic glucose output and a decrease in glucose uptake by peripheral tissues such as muscle. The resulting hyperglycaemia with glucosuria leads to a depletion of fluid and electrolytes and a fall in the rate of renal perfusion. There is simultaneous increase in lipolysis and mobilisation of fatty acids from adipose tissue to the liver, where they are broken down to fatty acyl-CoA and converted to ketone bodies (acetoacetate, acetone and β-hydroxybutyrate). An increase in circulating levels of β-hydroxybutyric acid reduces blood pH, leading to metabolic acidosis. There is a significant loss of fluid and electrolytes. Acidosis is aggravated further by progressive dehydration and impairment of renal excretion of ketone bodies. The effectiveness of pH-dependent enzyme systems is reduced at pH <7.0. If untreated, ketoacidosis leads to death.

The three biochemical indicators of ketoacidosis are hyperglycaemia, ketonaemia and acidosis. Ketoacidotic patients require hospital management, the principles of which include replacement of fluid and electrolyte losses, restoration of the acid–base balance, replacement of insulin, replacement of energy losses with glucose and identification of the underlying cause of ketoacidosis.[1]

Causes of diabetic ketoacidosis include undiagnosed type 1 diabetes or an inadequate dosage of exogenous insulin. It can also be triggered by the stress of an illness such as an infection. The requirement for insulin increases during stress. It is common for type 1 diabetic patients to omit insulin because they are unable to eat due to nausea or vomiting. Diabetic patients should be made aware that the blood glucose control can deteriorate rapidly during intercurrent illness and that their insulin dosage may need to be increased. The calorie intake also needs to be maintained to match the insulin dosage. Liquid forms of carbohydrate may be more appropriate if the patient is feeling sick (see Management Focus, p. 35).[2,3]

Non-ketotic hyperosmolar coma

Non-ketotic hyperosmolar coma is a condition that is characteristic of uncontrolled type 2 diabetes. It is characterised by a marked increase in blood glucose (usually >30 mmol/L) and severe dehydration, but without significant ketones or acidosis. The majority of cases of non-ketotic hyperosmolar coma occur in older people with type 2 diabetes. Symptoms of hyperglycaemia often develop insidiously and have often been present for several weeks.

This condition represents the other end of the spectrum of the biochemical processes involved in ketoacidosis, as there is sufficient endogenous insulin to inhibit hepatic ketogenesis. Relative insulin deficiency leads to an increase in hepatic glucose output and a decrease in glucose uptake by peripheral tissues such as muscle and adipose tissue. The resulting hyperglycaemia with glucosuria leads to a depletion of fluid and electrolytes and a fall in the rate of renal perfusion. Extreme dehydration and hyperosmolality leads to coma and death.

Clinical symptoms of dehydration and hyperosmolality include stupor or coma with an increased risk of stroke, myocardial infarction and arterial insufficiency in the lower limbs. Principles of management include monitored rehydration with sodium chloride solutions and administration of insulin. Non-ketotic hyperosmolar coma occurs in previously undiagnosed diabetes and may be related to age. Dehydration is more common in the elderly who experience thirst less acutely and mild renal impairment can lead to an increase in loss of fluid and electrolytes. Trigger factors include intercurrent illness and concurrent medication such as thiazide diuretics and steroids (see Management Focus, p. 29).[1]

Patients with type 2 diabetes should be made aware that their blood glucose control can deteriorate rapidly during an intercurrent illness and that they may require insulin. Maintaining an adequate fluid intake (to avoid dehydration) is essential, but inappropriate consumption of large quantities of sugar-containing drinks such as *Lucozade* (which can also precipitate non-ketotic hyperosmolar coma) should be avoided (see Management Focus below).[2,3]

Hypoglycaemia

Hypoglycaemia is a major cause of anxiety in patients and their relatives; it is the most common complication of insulin therapy and is also a common complication with the longer-acting sulphonylureas such as chlorpropamide and glibenclamide in elderly patients in a poor state of nutrition. Hypoglycaemic unawareness can occur in longstanding diabetic patients who have defects in secretion of counter-regulatory hormones such as glucagon and adrenaline, which have a role in the prevention of hypoglycaemia under normal physiological conditions. Hypoglycaemic unawareness can also occur in patients on intensive

MANAGEMENT FOCUS

Patient information on illness rules (sick day management)[2]

- Continue with the antidiabetic therapy (tablets or insulin) – insulin therapy should never be stopped
- Increase the frequency glucose monitoring (blood or urine)
- Adjust therapy according to previously arranged schedule (e.g. as discussed with the diabetic team)
- Continue carbohydrate intake (in a liquid form if necessary)
- Increase the amount of fluid intake (but caution with drinks with a high sugar content, particularly in the elderly)
- Consult GP promptly if the illness persists and the high glucose levels (blood or urine) continue, particularly if associated with vomiting

insulin therapy whose blood glucose concentrations have been lowered to normal or near-normal levels.[4]

Definition

Hypoglycaemia is clinically defined as the presence of symptoms associated with subnormal blood glucose levels, but there is no general agreement about which level of glucose defines hypoglycaemia. A classification of the severity of hypoglycaemia according to blood glucose concentration has been provided in some US sources as:[5]

- <50 mg/dL (<2.8 mmol/L): symptoms may or may not be present.
- <40 mg/dL (<2.2 mmol/L): symptoms usually present.
- <20 mg/dL (<1.1 mmol/L): associated with seizures and coma.

This definition of hypoglycaemia is considered to be dangerous in clinical terms as cognitive abnormality has been found to occur at a blood glucose level of about 3.0 mmol/L. Hypoglycaemic unawareness develops if blood glucose levels frequently fall below 3.0 mmol/L, and can be reversed by reducing the number of hypoglycaemic episodes. In clinical terms, the lower limit of blood glucose levels to prevent hypoglycaemic coma is considered to be about 4.0 mmol/L.[6]

Signs and symptoms

Symptoms vary, but tend to follow a constant pattern in individuals. They can be divided into two broad categories: (i) 'adrenergic' symptoms associated with catecholamine release; and (ii) 'defective nervous system' symptoms caused by low blood glucose levels. The stages of hypoglycaemia can be grouped according to symptoms (see Adverse Effects Focus, p. 37).

Management

Most patients have a tendency to over-treat hypoglycaemic reactions by consuming large quantities of quick-acting carbohydrate such as fruit juice. This action usually results in hyperglycaemia. Consumption of 10–20 g (or equivalent; see Management Focus, p. 38) of quick-acting carbohydrate is usually sufficient to treat most hypoglycaemic reactions. If after 15 min the blood glucose levels remain low, a further 10–20 g of quick-acting carbohydrate may be ingested. If a meal is not scheduled within the next 1–2 h, a small snack consisting of complex carbohydrate

Stages of hypoglycaemia classified according to symptoms[4,5]

Mild: 'Adrenergic' symptoms including anxiety, sweating, tremor, palpitations, feeling of hunger.
Action: Patients can help themselves by immediately consuming 'quick-acting' carbohydrate followed by complex carbohydrate (see Table 6.1, pp. 60–61).

Moderate: 'Defective nervous system' symptoms such as blurring of vision, confusion, intense hunger, severe headache, inability to accept advice and occasionally aggressive behaviour.
Action: Patient requires help but is not unconscious. Placing honey or sugar gel, *Hypostop*, onto gums may help. Once symptoms have subsided, the patient can eat complex carbohydrate (see Table 6.1, pp. 60–61).

Severe: Coma or convulsions.
Action: Patient needs to be placed in the recovery position and requires medical help. Glucagon*, if available, may help to reverse hypoglycaemia but intravenous glucose (dextrose) may be needed.

Nocturnal hypoglycaemia: Restless sleep or nightmares, profuse sweating, morning headache or 'hangover'. However, some patients do not experience any symptoms and high blood glucose levels before breakfast may be the only indicator of nocturnal hypoglycaemia.
Action: Check blood glucose levels at bedtime. Extra carbohydrate should be consumed if pre-bedtime blood glucose levels are below 6.0 mmol/L. High evening insulin dosage or peak action of the insulin in the middle of the night in patients who take intermediate-acting insulin before an evening meal can cause nocturnal hypoglycaemia. Adjustment in the evening dosage of insulin may be necessary if pre-bedtime blood glucose levels are consistently below 6.0 mmol/L over several days.

* Note. Glucagon is not suitable for treating hypoglycaemia in type 2 diabetic patients as these patients have reserves of endogenous insulin. Glucagon can stimulate insulin release and make the hypoglycaemia worse.

or protein should provide a continual source of glucose until the next scheduled meal.[5,7]

Causes

The risk of hypoglycaemia is highest before meals and at night. Hypo-glycaemic events may be caused by a variety of factors (see Adverse Effects Focus, p. 38). Hypoglycaemia can be avoided if patients and their carers have been adequately educated to monitor blood glucose levels

MANAGEMENT FOCUS

Food sources which provide 10 g (≡ one exchange) of carbohydrate	
Sugar (sucrose):	10 g (two teaspoonfuls)
Milk:	200 mL (one glass)
Unsweetened fruit juice:	100 mL
Soup:	200 mL (one cup)
Lucozade:	60 mL (four tablespoonfuls)

ADVERSE EFFECTS FOCUS

Causes of hypoglycaemia in diabetic patients

- Irregular eating habits
- Content of the diet
- Unusual level of exercise (see p. 39)
- Excessive alcohol intake (see p. 42)
- Variation in the injection site for insulin (see p. 83)
- Problems with blood glucose monitoring due to visual impairment or incorrect measuring technique (see Glucose Monitoring Focus, p. 49)
- Hypoglycaemic unawareness
- Delayed gastric emptying time (gastroparesis)
- Excessive dosage of insulin or sulphonylurea
- Recent changes in antidiabetic therapy
- Effect of other concurrent drug therapy
- Effect of concurrent use of complementary medicines

and to take appropriate measures when any changes in therapy or daily routine are made, or if the patient is unwell. Patients on insulin should understand the need for insulin and the duration of effect and peak times of insulin action with their individual insulin regimen. Meals should be taken at appropriate times to coincide with insulin action. Short-acting insulins can be taken 20–30 min before eating. It is essential that food is taken on a regular basis if twice-daily biphasic insulin is used, as the intermediate component of the mixture may lead to hypoglycaemia if a meal is delayed.[5]

Other conditions

People with diabetes are at risk for psychological disturbance resulting from being diagnosed as having diabetes and the likely impact of this diagnosis on their lifestyle. The risk of clinical depression is also high in people with diabetes. Up to 20% of people with diabetes suffer from depressive disorders. Depression can have a deleterious effect on the ability of the person with diabetes to manage their condition appropriately. Some people with diabetes develop anorexia nervosa, injection and needle phobias, and obsessional disorders.

People with diabetes and good glycaemic control are not more prone to infections than are non-diabetic individuals. However, susceptibility to infections (skin, urinary tract, lungs) is increased in diabetic patients with poor glycaemic control. Other common conditions in people with diabetes include soft tissue conditions (frozen shoulder, trigger finger, and diabetic hand syndrome) and skin conditions (granuloma annulare and necrobiosis lipoidica diabeticorum). There is an association between soft tissue conditions and poor glycaemic control.[3,8]

Exercise

Exercise increases energy consumption, and under normal physiological conditions this increase in requirement for energy is met by an increase in utilisation of glucose (from the breakdown glycogen in muscle and glycogenolysis and gluconeogenesis in the liver) and free fatty acids (from breakdown of triglycerides in adipose tissue). Blood glucose concentrations are maintained within the normal range through the action of counter-regulatory hormones such as glucagon and catecholamines.

Exercise is a fundamental component of diabetes management and it is therefore important that diabetic patients exercise regularly. The benefits of exercise in diabetes mellitus include: (i) improved glycaemic control due to increased insulin sensitivity and glucose tolerance; and (ii) reduction in cardiovascular risk factors due to an improvement in blood lipids profile, blood pressure and cardiovascular fitness and enhancement of body weight loss in obese diabetic patients. It is important that individual diabetic patients are assessed for, and are aware of, the risks associated with exercise before embarking on any exercise programme. Risks include:

- Immediate and prolonged hypoglycaemia (due to enhanced uptake of glucose by tissues induced by exercise).
- Exacerbation of hyperglycaemia and possible development of ketosis (if exercise is undertaken when in a state of insulin deficiency).
- Exacerbation of microvascular diabetic complications with some types of strenuous exercise (e.g. jarring exercise or exercise which involves moving

the head below the waist may precipitate haemorrhage or retinal detachment in patients with active proliferative retinopathy).

Inappropriate exercise can also lead to myocardial arrhythmias, ischaemia or infarction in diabetic patients with existing coronary artery disease or autonomic neuropathy. Diabetic patients with peripheral neuropathy may have a loss of sensation in their feet and therefore should avoid repetitive weight-bearing exercise as this can lead to ulceration and fractures (see pp. 17–18).[5,9]

Type 1 diabetes

Exercise can induce hyperglycaemia or hypoglycaemia depending on the degree of glycaemic control, the timing of insulin administration and food intake. The importance of regular glucose monitoring and adjustment of carbohydrate intake should be emphasised to the patient, as exercise alters both glucose metabolism and insulin absorption.

Hypoglycaemia can occur during, immediately after, or up to 15 h after exercise. It may result from an increase in insulin sensitivity, repletion of liver and muscle glycogen stores or peak action of intermediate-acting insulin and is more likely to occur if exercise is taken in the afternoon rather than the morning. Symptoms of hypoglycaemia may not be apparent during exercise. Hypoglycaemia can be avoided if the patient can acquire the knowledge and self-management skills to adjust insulin dosage and carbohydrate intake according to the following factors:

- Previously measured metabolic response to exercise.
- The planned duration and intensity of exercise.
- The insulin dosage regimen.
- The blood glucose concentration at the start of the exercise period.

Patients are then able to perform all levels of exercise, provided that they do not have diabetic complications (see above) and have good glycaemic control. The general recommendations for exercise in type 1 diabetic patients[9] are that tests for blood glucose levels should be carried out before, during (if individual response to exercise unknown) and after exercise. Pre-exercise fasting blood glucose levels of >16.7 mmol/L (300 mg/dL) or >13.9 mmol/L (250 mg/dL) with ketosis indicate insulin deficiency, and exercise should be postponed until glycaemic control is regained. If the pre-exercise glucose level is <5.6 mmol/L (100 mg/dL),

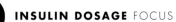

INSULIN DOSAGE FOCUS

> **Types of adjustments in insulin dosage and carbohydrate intake which may be necessary for type 1 diabetic patients before exercise**
>
> ***Exercise anticipated but insulin dose not injected.*** An adjustment of the insulin dosage may be necessary (e.g. reduction of 30–35% for intermediate-acting insulin and 50–65% for short-acting insulin). Exact adjustments can only be determined individually with blood glucose monitoring and the observed responses to different forms and levels of exercise. Vigorous exercise should not be undertaken unless the blood glucose level is within the range of 5.6–11.1 mmol/L and there is no sign of ketosis.
>
> ***Short-acting (e.g. soluble insulin) already injected.*** Advisable to avoid strenuous activity for up to 4 h to avoid the peak action insulin coinciding with the exercise. However, this is not necessary for patients on multiple injection therapy who inject small doses of short-acting insulin, adjusted according to results of blood glucose tests, three times daily before meals. In order to avoid hypoglycaemia from unplanned exercise, supplemental complex carbohydrate (e.g. 20–30 g depending on results of blood glucose tests) may be taken before and possibly during prolonged activity. There may be a requirement for additional food intake at the next meal.

then extra carbohydrate should be consumed in order to avoid hypoglycaemia (see Insulin Dosage Focus, above). A supply of carbohydrate-based food should be kept readily available during and after exercise (see Management Focus, p. 38).

Type 2 diabetes

Exercise generally decreases insulin resistance and reduces blood glucose concentrations in type 2 diabetic patients, but symptomatic hypoglycaemia is uncommon. Moderate, regular exercise is highly recommended for patients on diet-only or diet and oral antidiabetic therapy, particularly because of the effect of exercise in reducing cardiovascular risk factors. However, an assessment of cardiovascular fitness (e.g. a treadmill stress test) before embarking on an exercise programme is recommended. Regular, moderate exercise is also desirable in patients on insulin therapy, but these patients should be advised to take additional precautions such as increased food intake, delayed administration of insulin or reduced dosage of insulin, in order to avoid hypoglycaemia (see under type 1 diabetes, above).

Alcohol

Consumption of alcohol can cause hypoglycaemia in diabetic individuals as it impairs the body's ability to recover from hypoglycaemia by inhibiting hepatic gluconeogenesis. Alcohol intake can potentiate hypoglycaemia, and therefore should always be consumed with food. It may also reduce hypoglycaemia awareness. Glucagon treatment is less effective in alcohol-induced hypoglycaemia.

If blood glucose levels are well controlled, a moderate intake of alcohol with food does not usually cause any problems. Diabetes UK recommends a maximum daily intake of three drinks (1 drink: approximately 250 mL (half-pint) of beer or 23 mL of spirits). The calorific value of alcohol should be taken into consideration for those diabetic patients who are trying to lose weight, as alcohol yields a high amount of energy. The recommendation is for substitution of alcohol calories for fat exchanges (1 alcoholic beverage = 2 fat exchanges) or fat calories calculated as part of the total calorie intake (see Chapter 6). Excess alcohol can cause weight gain, high blood pressure and, in those taking sulphonylureas or insulins, can make hypoglycaemia more severe. Alcohol is best consumed with or after food.

Smoking

Smoking should be actively discouraged, as it is associated with an increased risk for development of diabetic complications such as proteinuria, foot problems and cardiovascular disease (see Chapter 3). Diabetic patients who smoke require more insulin than non-smokers, and smoking may also affect the absorption of insulin after subcutaneous injection. Patients on insulin should be informed that their insulin requirements may change if they are attempting to give up smoking or change their smoking habits.

Driving

Care should be taken to avoid hypoglycaemia while driving. The person with diabetes may be charged with driving under the influence of drugs and lose their licence if an accident is attributable to a hypoglycaemic episode. Simple precautions include checking blood glucose before the journey, stopping immediately if symptoms of hypoglycaemia develop, and always having readily available a source of rapidly absorbed carbohydrate such as glucose-containing drinks or tablets (see Management Focus, p. 38).[10]

Travel

Hypoglycaemic episodes when travelling long distances can be avoided by forward planning and taking a few simple precautions. If travelling on a long-haul flight, established regimens should not be altered during the flight. It is best to keep 'home time' for insulin and meals for journeys up to 8 h. For journeys longer than 8 h, advice about adjusting the regimen should be sought from the diabetes team. For those with a history of hypoglycaemia, a supply of glucagon carried by a travelling companion who knows when and how to administer it should be considered as a precautionary measure. Insulin and any other medication should be carried in the hand luggage along with some quick-acting carbohydrate (e.g. glucose-containing drinks or tablets). The essential items for air travel for people with diabetes treated with insulin include equipment (insulin vials or cartridges, syringes and needles or pens and needles, lancets, blood glucose meter and testing strips, urine ketone strips and spare batteries and blood testing meter), documents (diabetes identity card/bracelet, blood glucose monitoring diary, letter from doctor stating that the person has diabetes and details of treatment plus the necessity for carrying needles, syringes, etc.), treatment for hypoglycaemia (fast-acting carbohydrates such as glucose tablets/drinks and slow-acting carbohydrates such as biscuits and cereal bars), and fluids (bottled water or other glucose-free drinks). It is important that the insulin is kept cool, for example by keeping it in a 'cool bag' or a Thermos flask while travelling, and storing it in a refrigerator whenever possible.[10–12]

Vaccination

Infections can cause glycaemic control to deteriorate and increase the risk of diabetic ketoacidosis or hyperosmolar non-ketotic coma. People with diabetes are at risk of complications that may arise from infections such as influenza and pneumococcal pneumonia. Vaccination against influenza in people aged over 60 years and pneumococcal pneumonia in people aged over 65 is recommended. Vaccination in younger people with diabetes may be appropriate particularly if other risk factors such as cardiovascular or respiratory disease are present. Vaccination for influenza is needed on an annual basis, whereas for pneumococcal pneumonia it is only necessary once every 10 years.[13]

Complementary/alternative medicines

See Chapter 6, Dietary supplements.

References

1. Kumar P J, Clark M L (eds). *Clinical Medicine*, 2nd edition. London: Bailliere Tindall, 1990: 832–872.
2. British Diabetic Association. *Recommendations for the Management of Diabetes in Primary Care*. Diabetes Services Advisory Committee, British Diabetic Association, 1993.
3. Department of Health, National Service Framework for Diabetes: Standards 2002. Supplementary information. www.doh.gov.uk/nsf/diabetes (last accessed November 2002).
4. Nattrass M (ed.). *Malin's Clinical Diabetes*, 2nd edition. London: Chapman & Hall, 1996.
5. Koda-Kimble M A, Young L Y (eds). *Applied Therapeutics: The Clinical Use of Drugs*, 5th edition. Vancouver, Washington: Applied Therapeutics Inc., 1992: Chapter 72.
6. Mokan M, Mitrakou A, Veneman T, *et al.* Hypoglycaemia unawareness in IDDM. *Diabetes Care* 1994; 17: 1397–1403.
7. Diabetes in practice: Hypoglycaemia. Fact sheet 25. *Diabetes Update*. Summer 2002. Diabetes UK
8. Larkin J G. Musculoskeletal conditions in diabetes – multiple manifestations of one connective tissue process? *Mod Diabetes Management* 2002; 3: 8–11.
9. American Diabetes Association Position Statement. Diabetes mellitus and exercise. *Diabetes Care* 1998; 21 (Supplement 1): S40–S44.
10. Hillson R. *Practical Diabetes Care*. Oxford: Oxford University Press, 1996.
11. Anonymous. Advising patients about air travel. *Drug Ther Bull* 1996; 34: 30–32.
12. McAulay V. Diabetes and air travel. *Mod Diabetes Management* 2002; 3: 9–12.
13. Diabetes UK Care Recommendation. Influenza and Pneumococcal Pneumonia vaccinations. www.diabetes.org.uk/infocentre/carerec/vaccine.htm (last accessed December 2002).

5

Monitoring glycaemic control

The monitoring of glycaemic control is considered to be the cornerstone of diabetes care as it forms the basis for the day-to-day management of the condition.

Blood glucose monitoring

Self blood glucose monitoring is recommended for patients on insulin. Patients can routinely monitor their own blood glucose (whole blood, capillary) levels at home using blood glucose test strips and meters (see Table 5.1).[1] Ideally, most blood test results should be within the normal range (fasting ~5.0 mmol/L; post-prandial <10.0 mmol/L). It is important that an individual target range, which balances the long-term risks of hyperglycaemia against the risk of hypoglycaemia, has been agreed with the patient.[2]

If used appropriately, self blood glucose monitoring can help diabetic patients treated with insulin to take control of their diabetes. The results give an immediate indication of glycaemic control, allowing patients to make appropriate adjustments in their diet or insulin dosage. Individual plans for routine monitoring, outlining when and how often the tests should be carried out, can be useful if reviewed regularly. The most useful test-times for assessing hyperglycaemia are before breakfast, mid-morning, and 2 h after the evening meal. Tests carried out before main meals and at bedtime will give an indication of the efficacy of the preceding insulin dose and will also detect any hypoglycaemia.[3] Measurement of blood glucose can be particularly useful during illness or when undertaking strenuous exercise or dietary changes. Patients should be made aware of the importance of recording any changes in diet and exercise and also any episodes of hypoglycaemia, illness or stress. An accurate and detailed record can provide useful information during evaluation of treatment.

Self blood glucose monitoring is unlikely to serve any useful purpose if the patient does not have a full understanding of the measurement technique and the purpose for which the measurement is being

Table 5.1 Home blood glucose tests

Test strips	Visual range (mmol/L)	Meter*	Meter range (mmol/L)	Reagents	Manufacturer
A. VISUAL READING ONLY					
Hypoguard Supreme Spectrum	2.2–27.8				Hypoguard
B. METER READING ONLY					
Active		Glucotrend and Accu-Chek Active	0.6–33.3		Roche Diagnostics
Advantage II BM Accutest	–	Accu-Chek Advantage Accutrend	0.6–33.3 1.1–33.3	Colorimetric strips impregnated with glucose, oxidase and chromogens	Roche Diagnostics
Compact Esprit Biosensor ExacTec	–	Accu-Chek Compact Esprit ExacTech	0.6–33.3 0.6–33.3 2.2–25.0	Sensor discs Biosensor strips impregnated with glucose oxidase	Roche Diagnostics Roche Diagnostics Bayer Diagnostics
GlucoMen Glucotide	–	GlucoMen Glyco Glucometer 4	1.1–33.3 0.6–33.3	Colorimetric strips impregnated with glucose, hexokinase, diaphorase and tetrazolium indicator Bayer Diagnostics	MediSense Menarini Diagnostics

			Reading range (mmol/l)	Strip chemistry	Supplier
Hypoguard Supreme		*Hypoguard Supreme*	2.2–27.7	Biosensor strips impregnated with glucose oxidase	Hypoguard
MediSense G2	–	*MediSense*	1.1–33.0		MediSense
MediSense Optimum		*MediSense Optium*	1.1–33.0		MediSense
MediSense Soft-Sense		*MediSense Soft-Sense*	1.7–25		MediSense
One Touch	–	*One Touch*	0.0–33.3	Colorimetric strips impregnated with glucose oxidase, peroxidase, chromogens	LifeScan
One Touch Ultra		*One Touch Ultra*	1.1–33.3		LifeScan
PocketScan		*PocketScan*	1.1–33.3		LifeScan
Prestige Smart System		*Prestige Smart System*	1.4–33.3		Diagnosys

C. VISUAL + METER READING (Colorimetric strips impregnated with glucose oxidase, peroxidase, chromogens)

				Supplier
BM Test 1-44	*Reflolux S*	1.1–44.0	0.5–27.7	Roche Diagnostics
Glucostix	*Glucometer GX*	1.1–44.0	2.0–22.0	Bayer Diagnostics
Medi-Test Glycaemic C	*Glycotronic C*	1.1–44.4	1.1–33.3	BHR Pharmaceuticals

* Blood glucose monitoring meters are not allowed on FP10. Meters may be purchased directly from the manufacturer or from Community Pharmacies. For a list of blood glucose meters currently available see www.diabetes.org.uk.

GLYCAEMIC CONTROL FOCUS

Reference values for blood glucose[2]

Blood glucose (mmol/L)	Good	Acceptable	Poor
Fasting	4.4–6.7	6.7–7.8	>7.8
Post-prandial	4.4–8.9	8.9–10.0	>10.0

The fasting plasma blood glucose value (normal range 3.3–5.6 mmol/L) gives a reliable indication of the prevailing glucose concentration in type 2 diabetes. In frail elderly patients, it may be advisable to maintain fasting plasma glucose levels ≥5.5 mmol/L in order to reduce the risk of hypoglycaemia.

The target values quoted are for plasma blood glucose. Whole-blood capillary glucose values (obtained from finger prick tests) tend to be 10–15% lower than plasma glucose values if the haematocrit level is normal. Extremes in haematocrit levels can affect the test results from home blood glucose measuring systems. In general, high haematocrit levels give low results and low haematocrit levels give high results, with the exception of *Glucotide* and *One Touch* systems where very low levels (below 25%) may also give low results due to seepage of plasma in the test area.[4]

undertaken. It can cause feelings of anxiety, frustration and helplessness in patients if they do not understand the significance of the results and the action (if any) that needs to be taken when blood glucose levels are outside their personal target range (see Glucose Monitoring Focus, pp. 49–50).

Urine glucose and ketone monitoring

Glucose

Self monitoring of urine glucose is routinely used to detect major hyperglycaemic episodes in patients who are unable or unwilling to undertake blood glucose monitoring or where normoglycaemia is not required. Tests are usually performed two or three times each week, either fasting (first or second void of urine) or post-prandial (usually after the evening meal). The target is to keep urine free from glucose, which indicates that the blood glucose concentration has not increased above the renal threshold.

Monitoring glycaemic control with urine glucose test strips is only useful in patients with a normal renal threshold for glucose corresponding to a plasma glucose concentration of 10 mmol/L. There is

GLUCOSE MONITORING FOCUS

Patient education for self blood glucose monitoring[4,5]

A. The meter

The patient should understand or know:

- When and how to calibrate the meter (most meters require calibration for each new pack of test strips, see point B below)
- The position of the battery and the indicator for a low battery
- Correct storage of the meter, particularly in relation to the temperature and the humidity specifications

B. The test strips

The patient should understand or know:

- Correct storage of the test strips (rapid deterioration occurs if the strips are exposed to air or moisture)
- Identification of the number, strip or 'chip' to be used for the calibration of the meter for that particular pack of test strips

C. The blood sample

Preparation of the materials (meter, test strip, lancet, tissue paper) for the blood test

For some older meters, the strips are placed into the machine after the strip has been 'developed' with a blood sample for a specified amount of time. Newer machines require the strip to be inserted into the machine before application of the blood and generally require a smaller sample of blood.

Procedure of washing hands and drawing the blood sample

1. Wash hands in warm water.
2. Make sure that your hands are properly dried otherwise the blood will not form a drop and this may make it difficult to apply the blood to the test strip.
3. Milk the finger from the base to increase the blood flow to the tip of the finger.
4. Use the lancet (or finger-pricking device) to lance the finger. The side of the finger is a suitable place. It is best to avoid the balls of the finger as most of the nerves are concentrated in this part of the finger.
5. Hold the finger below the heart with the lanced part facing downwards until enough blood is available.
6. Completely cover the pad on the test strip without touching the pad with your fingers (some new meters are more sensitive than others and an error indicator, such as 'Err' or 'Low', will appear if the pad is not covered completely or a slight pressure is applied accidentally).
7. Read, record and interpret the results.

continued overleaf

Glucose Monitoring Focus (continued)

D. Causes of unusual readings

- Strips are out of date or have not been stored properly
- Incorrect application of the blood sample to the test strip
- The blood is not being removed from the test strip within the specified time (generally for older meters)
- Meter requires cleaning, has low battery or has not been calibrated properly. Newer meters usually alert the user with an 'error' message
- Patient is dehydrated or in a hyperosmolar non-ketotic state
- Patient possibly has a low or a high haematocrit value (see Glycaemic Control Focus, p. 48)
- Possible interference from other medication (see Glucose Monitoring Focus, p. 53)
- The test is being performed in conditions which are outside the temperature and humidity specifications for the meter

considerable variation in renal threshold between individuals. The renal threshold may be substantially increased in people with longstanding diabetes (which may result in an underestimation of blood glucose), whereas the renal threshold tends to be low or variable in children and pregnant women (which may result in an overestimation of blood glucose). In elderly patients who have a tendency to have a high renal threshold, glucosuria may be undetected unless the blood glucose value exceeds 15 mmol/L. The test results are also affected by fluid intake. A negative urine glucose test result is of limited value since it does not indicate specifically whether the patient has normal blood glucose levels, is moderately hyperglycaemic, or is hypoglycaemic. The major limitation is that urine glucose tests are not suitable for detecting any hypoglycaemic episodes in patients on insulin or sulphonylurea therapy.[6,7]

Ketones

Monitoring for ketones in the urine is an important part of management of type 1 diabetic patients. It is also useful for all diabetic patients during periods of acute illness such as an infection, stress or gastrointestinal disturbances. The presence of ketone bodies in the urine of a diabetic patient may indicate the need for change in therapy or impending or established ketoacidosis, which requires immediate medical attention (see pp. 33–34).

The ketone bodies, β-hydroxybutyric acid, acetoacetic acid and

Table 5.2 Urine glucose and ketone tests

Product name	Test form	Manufacturer
GLUCOSE TESTS		
Clinistix	Reagent strips impregnated with glucose oxidase, peroxidase and o-tolidine. For screening for glycosuria only. Not suitable for self-monitoring	Bayer Diagnostics
Clinitest	Copper reagent solution tablets with urine testing kit	Bayer Diagnostics
Diabur-Test 5000	Reagent strips: glucose oxidase, peroxidase, tetramethylbenzidine	Boehringer Mannheim Diagnostics
Diastix	Reagent strips: glucose oxidase, peroxidase, potassium iodide. Requires accurate timing of 30 seconds	Bayer Diagnostics
Medi-Test Glucose	Reagent strips: glucose oxidase, peroxidase, o-tolidine	BHR Pharmaceuticals
KETONE TESTS		
Acetest	Nitroprusside reagent tablets	Bayer Diagnostics
Ketostix	Reagent strips: sodium nitroprusside, glycine, phosphate buffer	Bayer Diagnostics
Ketur	Reagent strips: sodium nitroprusside, glycine, alkaline buffer	Boehringer Mannheim Diagnostics

acetone, are the breakdown products of fatty acids. β-Hydroxybutyric acid forms the highest proportion (approximately 75%). Urine ketone testing strips use the nitroprusside reaction to produce a purple colour in the presence of ketones (see Table 5.2). Glycine is required for the detection of acetone. Urine ketone levels are affected by the urine volume and concentration.[6]

Glycated haemoglobin (glycosylated haemoglobin, GHb, HbA$_{1c}$, HbA$_1$)

The glycated haemoglobin test measures the fraction of haemoglobin that is irreversibly bound to glucose (usually HbA$_{1c}$). This reaction occurs more readily as blood glucose increases above normal, and the measurement of HbA$_{1c}$ concentration in venous blood provides an indication of the level of glycaemic control over the preceding 2–3 months (see Glycaemic Control Focus, below). A 1% increase in HbA$_{1c}$ corresponds to an average increase of 2.0 mmol/L in blood glucose.[6,10,11]

Fructosamine

The fructosamine test measures glycated serum proteins, and reflects glycaemic control over the previous 1–2 weeks.[10]

GLYCAEMIC CONTROL FOCUS

Glycated haemoglobin reference values[2]			
	Good	*Acceptable*	*Poor*
HbA$_1$ (normal 5.0–7.5%)	<7.5	7.5–8.7	>8.7
HbA$_{1c}$ (normal 4.0–6.0%)	<6.0	6.0–7.0	>7.0

These values should be used as a broad guideline only. The 'normal' range of glycated haemoglobin values varies between laboratories because of the lack of standardisation of the assay method. At present it is not possible to directly compare glycated haemoglobin values generated in different laboratories with any accuracy.[10] It is therefore very important that the 'normal' reference values for the particular laboratory where the tests are carried out are used when assessing patients' glycaemic control. The majority of clinical laboratories in England now use methods for estimating HbA$_{1c}$ that have been aligned to the method used in both the Diabetes Control and Complications Trial (DCCT) and UK Prospective Diabetes Study (UKPDS). The International Federation of Clinical Chemistry (IFCC) has developed a new reference method which measures 'true' HbA$_{1c}$ and all laboratories will be required to use IFCC standardised methods for estimating HbA$_{1c}$ from 2004.[11]

Drug interference with blood and urine tests

Drugs may interfere with the glucose oxidase test (used to measure blood and urine glucose) and copper reduction test (*Clinitest* used for measuring urine glucose). However there are only a few well-documented clinical reports of drug interference with glucose tests (see Glucose Monitoring Focuses, below and p. 54).[12–15]

   Older methods for blood glucose measurement used o-toluidine, or depended upon the detection of reducing substances in the blood. Newer methods use the enzyme glucose oxidase immobilised on electrodes. A current is generated when oxygen is released from the glucose molecule. The enzymes hexokinase and glucose dehydrogenase are also used in blood glucose assay systems (see Table 5.1). Blood glucose concentrations are quantified either by a colorimetric method or an electronic (biosensor) method. Urine glucose testing is based either on detection of reducing substances (such as glucose) in the urine through reduction of a copper salt to produce a colour change (see copper reduction test below) or oxidation of the glucose in the urine to produce a colour change (see glucose oxidase test below).

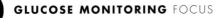

GLUCOSE MONITORING FOCUS

Drug interference with home blood glucose tests[13–15]

The following group of drugs may interfere with home blood glucose monitoring systems where the measurement of the glucose concentration is based on the glucose oxidase reaction.

Aspirin and salicylic acid: false low glucose results reported with in-vitro studies.

Paracetamol: false low glucose results reported with in-vitro studies.

Iodine: false apparent increases in blood glucose readings obtained when povidone–iodine swabs or tincture of iodine used instead of alcohol for cleansing fingers before testing. It is possible that the iodine, a strong oxidising agent, directly oxidises some colour indicators such as o-toluidine and tetramethylbenzidine on the reagent strip. The colour indicators in *Dextrostix* (e.g. 3,3'-dimethyl-4-4'-dimethylbiphenyl-dihydrochloride) do not appear to be affected.

Dopamine: the glucose oxidase reaction is inhibited by dopamine.

GLUCOSE MONITORING FOCUS

Drug interference with urine glucose and ketone tests[6,12]

Drug	CRT	GOT	Comments
URINE GLUCOSE			
GROUP A			There is evidence that this group of drugs interferes with *urine glucose tests*
Ascorbic acid (vitamin C)	–	✔	Possible false-positive results with intravenous administration. In-vitro studies indicate that 50–100 mg/dL of ascorbic acid is required to inhibit the reaction in urine samples containing 0.25% glucose. Higher concentrations of glucose require higher quantities of ascorbic acid
Antibiotics Cephalosporin Penicillin Aztreonam Imipenem	✔ ✔ ✔ ✔	– – – –	These β-lactam antibiotics do not have reducing properties but interfere with GOT tests possibly through the release of sulphur (on boiling) which reacts with copper ions to form insoluble coloured salts, e.g. copper sulphide (black)
Levodopa	✔	✔	Dose-related effect on urine glucose tests due to the strong reducing properties of the metabolite 3,4-dihydroxyphenylacetic acid
Salicylates (including aspirin)	✔	✔	Large chronic doses may produce false-positive results in both CRT and GOT. Interference appears to be due to a minor metabolite, gentisic acid
GROUP B			This group of drugs may interfere with *urine glucose tests* but documented evidence is limited
Chloral hydrate	✔	–	
Hyaluronidase	✔	–	
Nalidixic acid	✔	–	
Nitrofurantoin	✔	–	
p-Aminosalicylic acid	✔	–	
Probenecid	✔	–	
X-ray contrast media	✔	✔	

continued overleaf

Glucose Monitoring Focus (continued)

URINE KETONES

Ascorbic acid (vitamin C): False-negative readings have been reported after a large intake of ascorbic acid which makes the urine highly acidic. False-negative readings are also obtained when the test strip container has not been closed properly and the strips have been exposed to air for an extended period.

Captopril: Nitroprusside-containing reagents have been reported to give false-positive results. A similar effect is possible with other sulphydryl drugs.

CRT, Copper reduction test (includes reported interference with *Clinitest* only; reports with Benedict's solution have not been included); GOT, glucose oxidase test.

Glucose oxidase test

The colour change in this test is caused by two chemical reactions:

- Step 1: D-glucose is converted, by glucose oxidase, to D-glucuronic acid and hydrogen peroxide.
- Step 2: hydrogen peroxide, in the presence of peroxidase, oxidises a chromogen (indicator dyes) to produce a chromophore (a particular colour).

Drugs may interfere with these tests by inhibiting either glucose oxidase (step 1) or peroxidase (step 2) in the reaction (see Glucose Monitoring Focuses, pp. 53–55). There are no reports of false-positive results due to drugs, but cleansing agents such as hydrogen peroxide or sodium hypochlorite can cause such results if they are used for cleaning urine containers. The chromogen system (indicator dyes such as *o*-toluidine in *Clinistix*) varies between different products; therefore, drugs which affect step 2 may not affect all glucose testing systems in the same way.

Copper reduction test

Glucose reduces cupric sulphate (blue–green colour) to cuprous oxide (yellow to red–orange colour). Drugs or metabolites with reducing properties similar to glucose may inhibit this reaction and produce false-negative results. Some drugs can also cause confusion with the interpretation of the test by reacting with cupric sulphate to form other coloured compounds (see Glucose Monitoring Focus, p. 54 Group A: Antibiotics).

References

1. Anonymous. Meters for measuring blood glucose at home. *Drug Ther Bull* 1993; 31: 30–32.
2. British Diabetic Association. *Recommendations for the Management of Diabetes in Primary Care*. Diabetes Services Advisory Committee, British Diabetic Association, 1993.
3. Gallichan M. Self monitoring of glucose by people with diabetes: evidence-based practice. *Br Med J* 1997; 314: 964–967.
4. Koda-Kimble M A, Young L Y (eds). *Applied Therapeutics: The Clinical Use of Drugs*, 5th edition. Vancouver, Washington: Applied Therapeutics Inc., 1992: Chapter 72.
5. Montopoli T. Diabetes care. *Pharm Pract* 1998; 14: 62–71.
6. Goldstein D E, Little R R, Rodney A L, *et al*. Technical review: tests of glycaemia in diabetes. *Diabetes Care* 1995; 18: 896–909.
7. Anonymous. Should population screening be conducted for non-insulin dependent diabetes? *Diabetes Update* 1996; Winter: 4–5.
8. Department of Health National Health Service England and Wales. *Drug Tariff*. London: The Stationery Office, February 1997.
9. Frier B M. Glycated haemoglobin – is a 'single currency' desirable? *Diabet Rev Int* 1997; 6: 1–2.
10. Amiel S A, Gale E A M. Diagnostic tests in diabetes mellitus and hypo-glycaemia. In: Bouloux P-M G, Rees LH, eds. *Diagnostic Tests in Endocrinology and Diabetes*. London: Chapman & Hall, 1994: 187–214.
11. Department of Health. National Service Framework for Diabetes: Standards 2002. Interventions.
12. Rice G A, Galt K A. In vitro drug interference with home blood glucose measurement systems. *Am J Hosp Pharm* 1985; 42: 2202–2207.
13. Feingold K, Sater B, Engle B. Iodine-induced artifacts in home blood glucose measurements. *Diabetes Care* 1983; 6: 317.
14. Keeling A B, Schmidt P. Dopamine influence on whole blood glucose reagent strips. *Diabetes Care* 1987; 10: 532.
15. Rotblatt M D, Koda-Kimble M A. Review of drug interference with urine glucose tests. *Diabetes Care* 1987; 10: 105–110.

6

Dietary recommendations

The nutritional goals for people with diabetes are similar to those for a healthy diet in the non-diabetic population, with the aim of attaining and maintaining good control of blood glucose, lipids and blood pressure (see Chapter 3). The additional requirement for diabetic patients on insulin therapy is that the meal plans are individualised both in terms of the composition and the timing of meals and snacks in order to prevent excessive swings in blood glucose levels (see Management Focus, below).

The dietary recommendations for type 1 and type 2 diabetic patients are essentially the same, but the emphasis given to different components of the diet may vary according to individual circumstances.

Glycaemic index of foods

Different carbohydrates elicit different glycaemic responses, and these have been categorised in terms of the *glycaemic index* by comparison of the duration of hyperglycaemia elicited by different carbohydrates against the duration of hyperglycaemia elicited by an equivalent amount of glucose. The glycaemic index of various foods may be useful for selection of suitable foods for an individual diabetic patient.[2] For example, fruits and milk produce a lower glycaemic response than most

MANAGEMENT FOCUS

Goals of dietary therapy in management of diabetes mellitus[1]

- To maintain good glycaemic control in order to avoid diabetic emergencies and to prevent or delay the development of diabetic complications
- To attain and maintain reasonable body weight in type 1 diabetic patients and to preferably manage weight reduction in obese type 2 diabetic patients
- To attain and maintain optimal plasma lipid levels

MANAGEMENT FOCUS

Diabetes UK dietary recommendations for diabetic patients aiming for body mass index (BMI) of 22 kg/m²

- **Carbohydrate** 50–55% energy (composed of dietary fibre >30 g per day; sucrose or fructose <25 g per day)
- **Fat** 30–35% energy (composed of <10% saturated fatty acids; 10–15% monounsaturated fatty acids; <10% polyunsaturated fatty acids)
- **Protein** 10–15% energy

---

starches, whereas bread, rice and potatoes produce a glycaemic response similar to sucrose.[3] However, in practice, priority is given to the total amount of carbohydrate consumed rather than the source of carbohydrate in terms of the glycaemic index. The dietary components (i.e. carbohydrate, fat and protein) are expressed in terms of percentage of total energy intake (see Management Focus, above).[1]

Carbohydrates and fibre

Dietary carbohydrate consists of digestible carbohydrate which provides nutrition, and poorly digestible carbohydrate (fibre) which forms the roughage of the diet and facilitates intestinal motility and function (see Table 6.1). Following dietary intake of carbohydrate, blood glucose concentrations are raised above fasting level. The period of hyperglycaemia is kept to a minimum by the action of insulin, which promotes glucose uptake and utilisation by muscle and adipose tissue and storage as glycogen (a highly branched polysaccharide) in muscle and liver. Muscle glycogen is utilised exclusively by muscle, whereas liver glycogen is used to maintain blood glucose levels during the fasting state.

The general recommendation for diabetic patients is that the carbohydrate portion of the diet should mostly come in the form of complex carbohydrates, preferably from food high in natural dietary fibre or hydrolysis-resistant starch which is handled by the body in a similar way to soluble fibre (see Table 6.1). Cereal fibre and soluble fibre have a small hypoglycaemic effect in diabetic patients. Soluble fibre and leguminous fibre improve the blood lipids profile by reducing LDL-cholesterol and VLDL-cholesterol. Dietary fibre alone does not normalise diabetic abnormalities. Benefits are only seen when fibre is incorporated into an overall high-carbohydrate diet. However, the recommendation of a low-fat, high-carbohydrate diet for people with insulin resistance has been called into question. It has been suggested that the micronutrient composition of the diet may play an important role in fat deposition.[4]

Sucrose

The consumption of 'sugar' in modest amounts as part of the total carbohydrate content of the diet does not cause any major metabolic problems in either type 1 or type 2 diabetic patients. Restriction is recommended however, as overconsumption can lead to an increase in body weight. Low-calorie or low-sugar drinks do not offer a special advantage to diabetic patients. The only benefit such products offer is in reducing the risk of dental caries and, if used as a part of a low-calorie diet, for weight reduction. Insulin-treated patients are at risk of hypoglycaemia if they inadvertently consume reduced sugar foods either as a preventative measure or to treat symptoms of hypoglycaemia (see Adverse Effects Focus, p. 37).[5]

Sugar content of medicines

The advice from Diabetes UK is that for medicines used in small quantities for limited periods, the sugar content is unlikely to cause problems as it forms a small proportion of the carbohydrate content of the whole diet.[1] The sugar content of medicines may become significant in patients with poorly controlled diabetes or on low-calorie diets (10 mL syrup-based medicine $\equiv$ 35 calories). Sugar-free alternatives should be recommended if the medicine is for long-term use or the pharmaceutical form contains a lot of sugar (e.g. lozenges, but sugar-free versions are now available). Products containing hydrogenated glucose syrup (*Lycasin*) are not strictly 'sugar-free', as although hydrogenated glucose syrup is non-cariogenic, it is metabolised to glucose.[6] An information leaflet listing 'sugar-free' liquid medicines is available from the National Pharmaceutical Association (NPA).

Sugar in diabetic foods

Food products labelled as 'diabetic' usually contain sorbitol, fructose or xylitol (see Table 6.1). No significant difference has been found in blood glucose levels after the consumption of meals containing sucrose, fructose or sorbitol.[6] These sugars are calorifically equivalent to sucrose and are unlikely to offer any benefit in terms of weight reduction, even though sorbitol and xylitol are absorbed more slowly than glucose. Special 'diabetic' foods are usually more expensive and offer no advantage over low-calorie foods.

Table 6.1 Carbohydrates and sweeteners

Carbohydrate type	Other names	Composition	Sources and uses
MONOSACCHARIDES			
Glucose	Dextrose	Monosaccharide, also component of disaccharides, oligosaccharides	Glucose is the most abundant carbohydrate in food. It is the major physiological stimulus for insulin secretion from beta-cells
Fructose	Fruit sugar	Usually as disaccharides or or polysaccharides	Fruit and honey. About 75% sweeter than sucrose. No longer recommended as a sweetener in a diabetic diet as consumption of large amounts may have adverse effects on serum and LDL-cholesterol. Consumption of moderate amounts or as fruit does not appear to be a problem
Sorbitol		Derived from glucose	Fruits such as cherries, plums, apples and pears. Traditionally used as an alternative to sucrose in 'diabetic foods' as absorbed more slowly. It is rapidly converted to fructose in the body. Also used in ordinary foods such as sweets (increases shelf-life), soft drinks and wine (sequestrant), foodstuffs (reduces aftertaste of saccharin)
DISACCHARIDES			
Lactose	Milk sugar	Glucose + galactose	Cow's milk. Galactose is a constituent of polysaccharides and oligosaccharides in pectins, gums and mucilages

Sucrose	Sugar, cane sugar, beet sugar	Glucose + fructose	Honey
POLYSACCHARIDES			
Starch		Amylose (straight chain of glucose units) + amylopectin (branched glucose units)	Cereals, rice, potatoes
Fibre			Non-digestible polysaccharides found in vegetables, nuts, wheatbran and apples
OTHER SWEETENERS			
Aspartame		Aspartic acid + phenylalanine	Synthetic sweetener; negligible calorific value
Hydrogenated glucose syrup	*Lycasin*		Metabolised to glucose; non-cariogenic
Saccharin			Synthetic sweetener
Xylitol			Fruits and vegetables. Manufactured from xylan. Metabolised to glucose; non-cariogenic

Fat and triglycerides

Restriction of fat is advisable in both type 1 and type 2 diabetes because of the risk of cardiovascular complications. Lipid abnormalities are more common in type 2 diabetes (see pp. 21–27), and therefore a greater emphasis is placed on fat restriction (particularly saturated fat and cholesterol) in dietary advice for patients with type 2 diabetes. However, in type 2 diabetic patients, a low-fat diet (30% of total calories from fat) appears to be less effective in correcting dyslipidaemia and improving insulin sensitivity than a diet in which more calories are derived from monounsaturated fat. A diet with a higher monounsaturated fat content has been found to generate a proportional body fat loss from both upper and lower parts of the body, whereas a fibre-rich, high-carbohydrate, low-fat diet produced a disproportionate fat loss from the lower body and worsening of the fat distribution ratio. People with type 2 diabetes and insulin resistance may benefit from a diet rich in monounsaturated fat (e.g. from olive oil).[4]

Protein

A restriction of protein is likely to be beneficial in type 1 diabetes in modifying the progression of diabetic nephropathy (see pp. 13–16). It has been suggested that a higher protein content in the diet may be beneficial for weight loss as it results in lower loss of lean body mass but similar loss in body weight compared with a higher carbohydrate diet.[4]

Salt

The effect of sodium on blood pressure varies between individuals. The recommendations for sodium intake for people with diabetes are the same as for the non-diabetic population. The salt intake in people on a high-carbohydrate, high-fibre diet is not automatically reduced if the carbohydrate is ingested mainly in the form of bread and manufactured cereal foods. The recommendation is for salt intake to be limited to 3 g per day for those with hypertension, and 6 g per day for people without hypertension. The improvement in blood pressure is usually modest (a reduction of 1–2 mmHg on reducing salt intake from 10–12 g per day to 6 g per day), but it is associated with a marked reduction in the incidence of heart disease and stroke. A similar benefit may be obtained by increasing potassium intake in the form of fresh foods.[1,3] Salt intake is also associated with insulin resistance. Intake of sodium – either too high or too

MANAGEMENT FOCUS

Dietary advice for newly diagnosed diabetic patients[7]

- Have regular meals planned around starchy foods (e.g. bread, chapattis, potatoes, yam, pasta, plantin, rice, dahl, unsweetened potatoes)
- Have at least five portions of fruit and vegetables each day
- Reduce calorie intake if overweight or obese
- Reduce dietary intake of fat, particularly saturated fat
- Aim for low or moderate sucrose intake
- Increase intake of fibre, especially soluble fibre, and reduce dietary salt intake
- Aim for moderate alcohol intake (<10 drinks [glass of wine or half a pint of beer] per week for women and <20 drinks per week for men)

---

low – reduces insulin sensitivity. A severe reduction in dietary salt intake has been associated with an increase in serum lipids and insulin levels.[4]

All newly diagnosed patients should receive dietary advice from a dietician. However, some initial 'stop-gap' advice may be useful for patients who are waiting for more guidance from a dietician (see Management Focus, above).[7]

Dietary supplements

People with diabetes may be using dietary supplements as complementary or alternative forms of therapy for their diabetes, without informing the diabetes team. Clinical evaluations of a majority of these preparations have not been carried out in people with diabetes.

Ackee fruit (*Blighia sapida*)

Although two constituents of the unripe fruit of the ackee tree have been found to have potent hypoglycaemic properties, ingestion of the unripe ackee fruit has been associated with 'vomiting sickness' and a number of deaths in Jamaica. The hypoglycaemic constituents from the ackee fruit, known as the hypoglycins, are capable of inhibiting the oxidation of free fatty acids, leading to a depletion of liver glycogen and producing hypoglycaemia.[8]

Antioxidant vitamins

Abnormal endothelial function has been demonstrated in type 2 diabetes and to a certain extent also in type 1 diabetes. In diabetes mellitus, oxygen-derived free radicals impair endothelium-dependent vasodilatation. An improvement in endothelium-dependent vasodilatation by scavengers of oxygen-derived free radicals has been demonstrated in animal studies.[9] Agents such as vitamins C and E and a-carotene, which possess antioxidant properties, may prevent the oxidation of low-density lipoproteins and slow down atherogenesis. However, large randomised controlled trials in adults aged 40 to 80 years with coronary disease, other occlusive arterial disease or diabetes have found no significant reduction in 5-year mortality or incidence of cardiovascular events with antioxidant vitamins (vitamin E 600 mg, vitamin C 250 mg and beta-carotene 20 mg daily).[10]

Aloe vera

The dried sap of the plant has been shown to slightly reduce blood glucose levels, and topical application may help in wound healing.[8]

Biotin

Biotin is considered to be a vitamin B substance. It is an essential co-enzyme in fat metabolism and in other carboxylation reactions. It has been found to improve glucose metabolism in people on dialysis and type 2 diabetes.[4]

Burdock root

This contains inulin, and powdered burdock root has been found to reduce post-prandial hyperglycaemia after ingestion of a starch meal in people with diabetes.[8]

Fenugreek seeds

The main effect of fenugreek seeds – the reduction of blood sugar levels and improvement of glucose tolerance – is thought to be due to the fibre content of the seeds.[8]

Jerusalem artichoke (*Helianthus tuberosa*)

Jerusalem artichoke contains inulin, and has been found to slightly lower blood glucose levels after ingestion of high-fructose content meals in people with diabetes.[8]

Karela (*Momordica charantia*)

Common names for karela include bitter gourd, bitter melon, balsam pear and cundeamour. It produces a significant improvement in glycaemic control in type 2 diabetic patients when used as herbal medicine (fresh or dried), or when cooked and eaten as a part of a meal. The vegetable contains a peptide, polypeptide-p2, that has hypoglycaemic properties. Information on whether there is an increased risk of hypoglycaemia when used concomitantly (as a herbal medicine or food) with conventional hypoglycaemic agents is lacking.[11]

Garlic (*Allium sativum*)

Garlic has been shown to have a beneficial effect on blood lipids profile (reduced cholesterol and triglycerides and improved LDL/HDL ratio). The increase in blood lipids following a fatty meal has been reported to be prevented by garlic supplements. Other reported beneficial effects of garlic include a hypotensive effect (a reduction of 12–30 mmHg systolic and 7–20 mmHg diastolic blood pressure in patients with essential hypertension after regular ingestion of garlic), antithrombotic activity and hypoglycaemic effect. The mild blood glucose-lowering effect of garlic is thought to be due to the allylpropyldisulphide constituents.[8,12]

Ginseng

An 8-week-long Finnish study has reported that ginseng therapy elevates mood, improves physical performance and improves both fasting blood sugar and body weight in type 2 diabetic patients. Information on concomitant use with conventional antidiabetic drugs is lacking.[13]

Glucomannan

This is a dietary fibre which has been shown to reduce mean fasting glucose levels when taken as a dietary supplement for 90 days.[8]

Guar gum (Karaya gum)

Guar gum, a naturally occurring soluble fibre, slows down gastric emptying and carbohydrate absorption if ingested with a meal. It can reduce post-prandial increases in blood glucose if taken before a meal. Side effects include flatulence, abdominal bloating and diarrhoea. It is available as granules (*Guarem*), but is little used nowadays.

Gymnena

Gymnena inhibits the ability to taste bitter or sweet flavours, and this may lead to ingestion of fewer calories. Gymnena also has a hypoglycaemic effect.[8]

Magnesium

An association between magnesium deficiency and insulin resistance has been suggested, but no improvement in glycaemic control has been found in people with type 2 diabetes taking magnesium supplements.

Thioctic acid

Thioctic acid is also known as lipoic acid or alpha-liponic acid. Supplements of thioctic acid have been found to improve insulin sensitivity in people with diabetes.[4]

References

1. British Diabetic Association. Dietary recommendations for people with diabetes: an update for the 1990s. Compiled by the Nutrition Sub-Committee of the Professional Advisory Committee, British Diabetic Association. *Diabet Med* 1992; 9: 189–202.
2. Department of Health. National Service Framework for Diabetes: Standards 2002. www.doh.gov.uk/nsf/diabetes
3. American Diabetes Association Position Statement. Nutrition recommendations and principles for people with diabetes mellitus. *Diabetes Care* 1998; 21(Supplement 1): S32–S35.
4. Kelly G S. Insulin resistance: lifestyle and nutritional interventions. *Alternative Medicine Review* 2000; 5: 109–132.
5. Alain Li Wan Po. *Non-Prescription Drugs*, 2nd edition. Oxford: Blackwell Scientific Publications, 1990.
6. Lenner R A. Specially designed sweeteners and foods for diabetics – a real need? *Am J Clin Nutr* 1976; 29: 726–733.
7. Department of Health. National Service Framework for Diabetes: Standards 2002. Supplementary information. www.doh.gov.uk/nsf/diabetes
8. Gori M, Campbell R K. Pharmacy Update: Natural products and diabetes treatment. *The Diabetes Educator* 1998; 24: 201–208.
9. Hsueh W A, Law R E. Cardiovascular risk continuum: implications of insulin resistance and diabetes. *Am J Med* 1998; 105: 4S–14S.
10. Heart Outcomes Prevention Evaluation Study Investigators. Vitamin E supplementation and cardiovascular events in high-risk patients. *N Engl J Med* 2000; 342: 154–160.

11. Stockley I H. *Drug Interactions*, 4th edition. London: Pharmaceutical Press, 1996.
12. Newall C A, Anderson L A, Phillipson J D. *Herbal Medicines. A Guide for Health-Care Professionals*. London: Pharmaceutical Press, 1996: 129–133.
13. Sotaniemi E A, Haapakoski E, Rautio A. Ginseng therapy in non-insulin dependent diabetic patients. *Diabetes Care* 1995; 18: 1373–1375.

7

Pharmacotherapeutic interventions with antidiabetic drugs

There are six classes of drugs with different mechanisms of action currently available in the UK for the management of hyperglycaemia in diabetes mellitus (see Figure 7.1):

- Sulphonylureas and meglitinides (increase insulin secretion – see pp. 103–106 and pp. 129–130).
- Biguanides (metformin increases intracellular glucose metabolism and decreases hepatic glucose output – see pp. 113–114).
- Thiazolidinediones/peroxisome proliferator-activated receptor (PPAR)-γ-agonists (increase insulin sensitivity in skeletal muscle and adipose tissue – see pp. 123–125).
- Alpha-glucosidase inhibitors (acarbose reduces post-prandial hyperglycaemia by slowing down carbohydrate digestion – see pp. 119–120).
- Exogenous insulin (see pp. 79–83).

Type 1 diabetes

Exogenous insulin is the only option currently available for the correction of insulin deficiency in type 1 diabetes.

Type 2 diabetes

There are several pharmacotherapeutic options for management of hyperglycaemia in type 2 diabetes. These include use of sulphonylureas, meglitinides, metformin, acarbose, thiazolidinediones (PPAR-γ-agonists) and exogenous insulin either as monotherapy or combined in a stepwise fashion for better glycaemic control (see Management Focus, p. 71). The distinction between obese and non-obese type 2 diabetic patients is an important one and has implications on the management plan. The primary defect in obese patients is thought to be that of peripheral insulin resistance, whereas in non-obese patients the main problem may

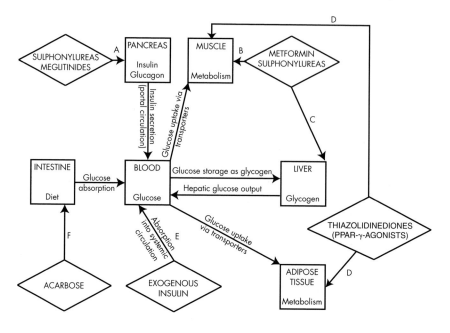

Figure 7.1 Schematic representation of targets for pharmacotherapeutic interventions for controlling hyperglycaemia in diabetes mellitus. (A) Stimulation of endogenous insulin secretion by sulphonylureas and meglitinides. (B) Potentiation of insulin action by metformin and possibly sulphonylureas. (C) Inhibition of hepatic gluconeogenesis and glycogenolysis resulting in reduced hepatic glucose output by metformin, and sulphonylureas (through action of insulin). This action contributes toward reducing fasting hyperglycaemia. (D) Increased insulin sensitivity through increased glucose uptake and glycolysis by thiazolidinediones (PPAR-γ-agonists). (E) Hormone replacement with exogenous insulin to compensate for the lack of insulin in diabetes mellitus. (F) Inhibition of polysaccharide digestion by competitive, reversible inhibitors of alpha-glucosidase enzymes such as acarbose leading to a reduction in post-prandial hyperglycaemic peaks.

be a defect in the insulin secretory mechanism.[1,2] A reduction in body weight reduces insulin resistance and improves glycaemic control in type 2 diabetic patients who are obese. These patients need to reduce their energy intake in order to reduce their body weight. If glycaemic control is poor on dietary therapy alone, the decision as to which antidiabetic drug the patient is initiated on depends upon the severity of the symptoms and the body mass index (BMI).

The United Kingdom Prospective Diabetes Study (UKPDS) was initiated in 1977 to determine whether aiming treatment to achieve

Stages of management of people with type 2 diabetes*

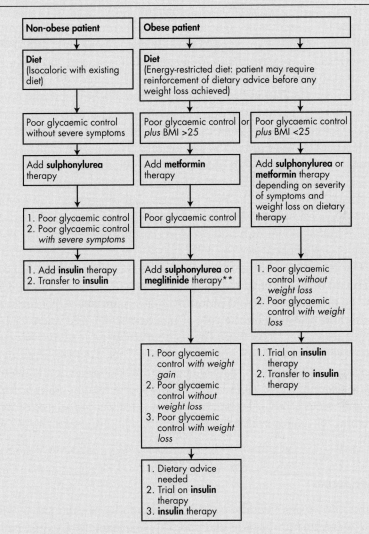

The thiazolidinediones (PPAR-γ-agonists), pioglitazone or rosiglitazone, should be considered in people who are not able to take metformin and sulphonylurea combination therapy. The combination of metformin plus a thiazolidinedione is preferred.

In addition to effects on blood glucose and body weight, the cardiovascular risk–benefit profile of the antidiabetic drug is an important factor in influencing the choice of antidiabetic drug for the management of type 2 diabetes.[3]

*Adapted from Watkins, P J. *Guidelines for good practice in the diagnosis and treatment of non-insulin dependent diabetes mellitus.*[4] and Royal College of General Practitioners Effective Clinical Practice Unit. Clinical Guidelines for Type 2 Diabetes, 2002.[5]

normal blood glucose levels (<6.0 mmol/L) prevents onset of microvascular and macrovascular diabetic complications (see Chapter 3), and also to compare advantages and disadvantages of different forms of treatment. Newly diagnosed type 2 diabetic patients were treated with diet alone for 3–4 months. Those in whom fasting blood glucose concentrations continued to be >6.0 mmol/L were randomised into three groups: (i) diet alone; (ii) diet with a sulphonylurea; and (iii) additional basal insulin (ultra lente). Obese patients were treated with metformin. Results of the UKPDS indicate that the difference in metabolic control of the different treatment groups is small (average values: diet group HbA_{1c} = 7.2%, oral antidiabetics or insulin group HbA_{1c} = 6.5%), and no differences were found in the rate of cardiovascular complications in different treatment groups.[6–8] However, the UKPDS has confirmed that intensive management of hyperglycaemia (i.e. maintenance of HbA_{1c} at approximately 7% over the first 10 years after diagnosis) substantially reduces the risk of microvascular complications in type 2 diabetes. Intensive management of blood pressure significantly reduces the risk of diabetic complications (see pp. 19–21).

The RCGP clinical guidelines for management of blood glucose[5] recommend that, on the initial diagnosis of type 2 diabetes, HbA_{1c} levels should be measured at 2- to 6-monthly intervals and the target for HbA_{1c} levels should be based on the risk of macrovascular and microvascular complications (see Chapter 3). The recommendation is to aim for target HbA_{1c} levels between 6.5 and 7.5% (DCCT & UKPDS aligned; see Glycaemic Control Focus, p. 52). Lower HbA_{1c} target levels are preferred for people with a significant risk of macrovascular complications, but higher HbA_{1c} target levels are necessary for people at risk of hypoglycaemia, for example elderly people with type 2 diabetes treated with insulin.[5]

Sulphonylureas

Sulphonylureas significantly lower both blood glucose and HbA_{1c} levels on initial treatment of newly diagnosed type 2 diabetic patients. Failure to control hyperglycaemia on initiating treatment with a sulphonylurea (primary failure) is usually due to the inappropriate use of a sulphonylurea in type 1 diabetes. In some patients, the hypoglycaemic effect of the sulphonylurea tapers off with continued treatment, with HbA_{1c} values returning to pre-treatment levels. This effect – referred to as 'secondary failure' – is thought to be a result of the progression of the disease rather than to reflect a loss in the effect of the sulphonylurea.

There is no widely accepted definition of 'secondary failure', and it is not known whether secondary failure is inevitable in all type 2 diabetic patients. It has been proposed that chronic stimulation of the islet beta-cells, particularly by long-acting sulphonylureas, causes premature beta-cell exhaustion and may also increase the output of immature beta-cell products such as proinsulin and split proinsulin, which in turn may increase atherogenesis. At this stage of the disease, secretion of the immature products of the beta-cell could be avoided by treating with insulin, which suppresses the 'sick' beta-cell. However, it is important to bear in mind that factors other than sulphonylurea failure may cause loss of glycaemic control. These include patient-related factors (dietary failure, stress, or intercurrent illness), disease-related factors (onset of type 1 diabetes, or increased insulin resistance) or other concurrent therapy-related factors (impaired absorption of sulphonylurea due to hyperglycaemia or concomitant use of drugs which impair glucose tolerance (see Management Focus, p. 29).

Meglitinides

The meglitinides (nateglinide, repaglinide) are used for regulating post-prandial hyperglycaemia because of their fast onset and short duration of action. This means that meglitinides may be taken shortly before a main meal. Repaglinide is licensed for use as monotherapy in people who are not overweight but their blood glucose levels increase over time. Both nateglinide and repaglinide are licensed for use in combination with metformin for people who are overweight and good glycaemic control is not being achieved with metformin alone (see pp. 129–130).[5]

Metformin

Metformin does not cause weight gain or hypoglycaemia in type 2 diabetic patients. It decreases both basal and post-prandial blood glucose levels after 2–6 weeks of treatment, and decreases HbA_{1c}, plasma insulin, total cholesterol, LDL-cholesterol and triglyceride levels, with a slight increase in HDL-cholesterol, after 3–4 months of treatment. Vascular effects of metformin include increased fibrinolytic activity and decreased sensitivity to platelet-aggregating agents. Intensive management of hyperglycaemia with metformin significantly reduces diabetes-related complications and mortality in obese patients.[8]

Approximately 5% of patients are not able to tolerate metformin therapy due to initial gastrointestinal side effects, and there is failure to improve glycaemic control in approximately 10% of patients (primary failure). Lower doses and more frequent assessments are recommended in the elderly.[9] The potential advantage of metformin not causing weight gain does not have major clinical significance in the elderly, who are often underweight. Progression of the disease in type 2 diabetic patients may lead to a loss of production of insulin by the beta-cell, which then leads to a deterioration in glycaemic control. As the mechanism of biguanide action does not involve direct stimulation of islet beta-cells, the production of immature beta-cell products is unlikely (see pp. 113–114). However, as metformin requires the presence of insulin to be effective, it may be necessary, at this stage of the disease, to transfer the patient onto exogenous insulin therapy.

Thiazolidinediones

Thiazolidinediones (PPAR-γ-agonists), pioglitazone and rosiglitazone, are licensed in the UK for use in combination with metformin or a sulphonylurea if metformin is not appropriate (see pp. 123–125).

Insulin

Insulin therapy is indicated in the type 2 diabetic patient who is symptomatic and losing weight. At this point it is likely that the pancreatic beta-cells have failed and that the patient is insulin-deficient. Insulin therapy can correct endogenous insulin deficiency and reduce blood glucose levels, which in turn reduces the toxic effects of chronic hyperglycaemia. In some type 2 diabetic patients, a trial with exogenous insulin therapy may be sufficient to improve endogenous insulin secretion so that the patient may be able to revert to oral antidiabetic therapy for glycaemic control.

The use of insulin therapy in type 2 diabetic patients with insulin resistance has been controversial as hyperinsulinaemia has been associated with atheroma-related diseases. The rationale behind using insulin therapy in type 2 diabetic patients who are insulin-resistant is based on the assumption that all cells are equally resistant and that hyperglycaemia is a biological indicator of insufficient insulin action. High plasma insulin concentrations are required to overcome this resistance to restore blood glucose concentrations to normal. The counter-argument is that all cells may not be equally resistant to the action of insulin. The harmful effect of excessive insulin on less resistant cells may increase the risk of coronary heart disease, for example by affecting the development of atheroma in the arterial wall and by the aggravation of hypertension. The suggestion that the increased risk of mortality from cardiovascular disease in diabetic patients is related to high levels of insulin rather than to hyperglycaemia is based on observations from epidemiological studies which show that a high fasting plasma insulin concentration is a risk factor for mycocardial infarction and other atheroma-related diseases. However, there is no direct evidence that insulin treatment affects the development of atheroma or hypertension,[10] and no evidence has been found of an increased risk of myocardial infarction in type 2 diabetic patients treated with insulin.[7]

Insulin therapy in the elderly

Several factors have to be taken into consideration before initiating insulin therapy in elderly patients. There may be problems, such as poor eyesight due to cataract formation, tremor and poor muscular co-ordination, which directly affect the patient's ability to inject the correct dose of insulin and monitor their blood glucose. Many elderly patients are not able to acquire new knowledge and to make the necessary changes to their lifestyle in order to look after themselves when on insulin therapy. These patients would have to rely on relatives or community care staff to take care of their insulin therapy, with the resulting loss of independence and self-esteem. The elderly are also more susceptible to hypoglycaemia, partly due to poor understanding and knowledge but also due to other physiological factors. Under normal physiological conditions, counter-regulatory hormones (glucagon, adrenaline, growth hormone and cortisol) are secreted in response to hypoglycaemia. These hormones counteract the action of insulin. An impairment in this counter-regulatory response or in insulin clearance increases the risk of severe hypoglycaemia, which can be fatal. In the elderly, both the counter-regulatory response and insulin clearance may be impaired. However, when considering the potential value of insulin therapy in the elderly, it is important that patients are treated as individuals and the decision is based on an assessment of the 'biological age' rather than the 'chronological age'. For example, a 75-year-old patient who is active, alert and physically fit would gain greater benefit than a 65-year-old patient who has had a cerebrovascular accident and is frail.[11]

Acarbose

Acarbose reduces post-prandial hyperglycaemia in type 2 diabetes, but does not appear to have a significant impact on fasting blood glucose levels and glycosylated haemoglobin concentrations (see pp. 119–120).[12]

Combination therapy in type 2 diabetes

Sulphonylurea plus metformin

This combination has been widely studied and is the most commonly used. Reductions in fasting blood glucose (25–30%) and glycated haemoglobin (20–30%) have been achieved in studies where metformin (1.5–2.5 g) has been added when sulphonylurea monotherapy has failed in type 2 diabetic patients. In these studies the doses of the sulphonylurea (both first and second generation; see Chapter 9, Table 9.1) were relatively high. The use of the combination of metformin and glibenclamide at lower doses in type 2 diabetic patients (with failure to control mild hyperglycaemia with diet alone) has shown no additive benefit when compared with monotherapy with either drug.[3] An interesting finding of the study (UKPDS 34) was the significant increase in diabetes-related death and all-cause mortality when metformin therapy was added to sulphonylurea therapy. It has been suggested that this may partly be due to the subgroup of patients studied who were on average 5 years older, more hyperglycaemic and less overweight, but that the effect requires further study.[8]

Sulphonylurea plus thiazolidinedione

See under metformin plus thiazolidinedione, below.

Sulphonylurea plus acarbose

In trials conducted in the US and Canada, a significant reduction in post-prandial hyperglycaemia, modest reductions in fasting plasma glucose concentration and a decrease in HbA_{1c} (0.5–1.0%) have been achieved when acarbose has been added, in progressively titrated doses, to sulphonylurea therapy. The incidence of hypoglycaemia and gastro-intestinal disturbances were not increased in comparison with monotherapy with either drug.[3]

Sulphonylurea plus insulin

This combination has been used in patients who show a partial response to sulphonylureas. A dose of an intermediate- or long-acting insulin (see Chapter 8, Table 8.1) is given at bedtime to reduce fasting hyperglycaemia, and the assumption is that this leads to an improvement in the sulphonylurea action during daytime.[3] The rationale for its use is that since sulphonylureas stimulate endogenous insulin secretion, lower doses of insulin are required for better glycaemic control. This is offset by the requirement for the patient to take both oral antidiabetic medication and insulin. The effect on glycaemic control is modest (expected reductions in HbA$_{1c}$ approximately 1.0–1.5%) and therefore the complexity of the treatment regimen may not be justified.

Metformin plus acarbose

Information on the use of this combination is lacking. There is a theoretical possibility that the frequency of gastrointestinal disturbances may be increased if these drugs are used in combination.[3] Acarbose affects the bioavailability of metformin (see p. 117).

Metformin plus meglitinides

See under meglitinides, above.

Metformin plus thiazolidinediones (PPAR-γ-agonists)

The thiazolidinediones (pioglitazone and rosiglitazone) are currently licensed for the use in oral combination therapy in management of patients with type 2 diabetes who have insufficient glycaemic control despite maximal tolerated dose of oral monotherapy with either metformin or a sulphonylurea. The recommendation is that thiazolidinediones be used in combination with metformin only in obese patients and in combination with a sulphonylurea only in patients who show intolerance to metformin or for whom metformin is contraindicated (see Management Focus, p. 71).[5]

Metformin plus insulin

There is very little information available on the use and effectiveness of this combination. The rationale for its use would be that in a poorly controlled obese patient, metformin would be expected to reduce the high requirement for insulin and also prevent weight gain.[13]

References

1. Alberti K G M M, Gries F A. Management of non-insulin-dependent diabetes mellitus in Europe: a consensus view. *Diabet Med* 1988; 5: 275–281.
2. Anonymous. Non-insulin-dependent diabetes mellitus (part 2). *MeRec Bull* 1996; 7: 29–32.
3. American Diabetes Association Consensus Statement. The pharmacological treatment of hyperglycaemia in NIDDM. *Diabetes Care* 1995; 18: 1510–1518.
4. Watkins P J. Guidelines for good practice in the diagnosis and treatment of non-insulin dependent diabetes mellitus. Report of a joint working party of the British Diabetic Association, The Research Unit of the Royal College of Physicians, and The Royal College of General Practitioners. *J R Coll Phys Lond* 1993; 27: 259–266.
5. Royal College of General Practitioners Effective Clinical Practice Unit. Clinical Guidelines for Type 2 Diabetes: Management of Blood Glucose, 2002. www.nice.org.uk (last accessed December 2002).
6. Wolffenbuttel B H R, van Haeften T W. Prevention of complications in non-insulin dependent diabetes mellitus (NIDDM). *Drugs* 1995; 50: 263–288.
7. UK Prospective Diabetes Study (UKPDS) Group. Intensive blood-glucose control with sulphonylureas or insulin compared with conventional treatment and risk of complications in patients with type 2 diabetes (UKPDS 33). *Lancet* 1998; 352: 837–853.
8. UK Prospective Diabetes Study (UKPDS) Group. Effect of intensive blood-glucose control with metformin on complications in overweight patients with type 2 diabetes (UKPDS 34). *Lancet* 1998; 352: 854–865.
9. Moorandian A D. Drug therapy of non-insulin-dependent diabetes mellitus in the elderly. *Drugs* 1996; 51: 931–941.
10. Turner R C, Holman R R. Insulin use in NIDDM. Rationale based on pathophysiology of disease. *Diabetes Care* 1990; 13: 1011–1019.
11. McDowell J R S, Gordon D. *Diabetes. Caring for Patients in the Community.* London: Churchill Livingstone, 1996.
12. Johnson A B, Taylor R. Drugs in focus: 19. Acarbose. *Prescribers' Journal* 1996; 36: 169–172.
13. Giugliano D, Quatraro A, Consoli G, *et al*. Metformin for obese, insulin-treated diabetic patients: improvement in diabetic control and reduction of metabolic risk factors. *Eur J Clin Pharmacol* 1993; 44: 107–112.

8

Insulins

Indications

Exogenous insulin is given as replacement therapy to compensate for the lack of endogenous insulin in type 1 diabetes and the relative lack of endogenous insulin (due to insulin resistance or a defect in the insulin release mechanism) in type 2 diabetes (see Chapter 7).

Mechanism of action

The basic metabolic defect in diabetes mellitus is that glucose cannot enter the cells, either because there is a lack of insulin (deficiency) or because the insulin that is present is ineffective (resistance). This defect can be managed by administration of exogenous insulin. Insulin decreases blood glucose concentrations by promoting glucose uptake from blood into cells where it has major effects on carbohydrate, lipid and protein metabolism. The key target tissues for insulin action are liver, skeletal muscle and adipose tissue, although insulin influences the function of most tissues. At the cellular level, insulin stimulates glycogen synthesis, lipid synthesis and glucose oxidation and simultaneously inhibits glycogenolysis, lipolysis and gluconeogenesis.[1]

Insulin molecule

Insulin, C-peptide and basic amino acids are released into the circulation together with some proinsulin in response to increases in blood glucose concentration above fasting level. Until recently, C-peptide was considered to be a by-product of insulin synthesis with little physiological significance. Recent research (in animals) indicates that it may have an important physiological role in maintaining vascular and neuronal function.[2]

The insulin molecule contains two polypeptide chains, chain A (21 amino acids) and chain B (30 amino acids), linked by two disulphide bridges (see Figure 8.1). Chain A has an additional disulphide bridge. The active site (residues 23–26, Gly-Phe-Phe-Tyr) of the hormone is

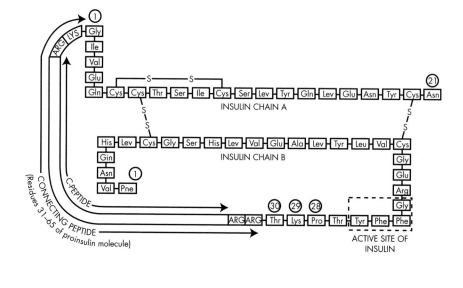

Figure 8.1 Schematic representation of proinsulin molecule highlighting the insulin part of the molecule.

located on the carboxy-terminal region of chain B. Mutations which affect the amino acid composition of the active site region affect biological activity of normal insulin. The solubility of insulin is less than that of proinsulin, which has a higher solubility because its hydrophobic region is masked by the connecting peptide part of the molecule. In the presence of zinc within the storage granules, endogenous insulin forms microcrystals of zinc–insulin hexamers. This crystalline state allows insulin to be stored in the most concentrated form and protects the molecule from further proteolytic cleavage. C-peptide is the 31-amino acid chain molecule remaining after cleavage of two pairs of basic amino acids from each end of the connecting peptide part of the proinsulin molecule.

Insulin secretion

Endogenous insulin secretion is affected by a wide range of physiological agents. The secretory response of the beta-cell to physiological stimuli occurs within seconds, requires the presence of calcium, and is controlled by fluctuations in extracellular concentrations of nutrients and hormones. The autonomic nervous system also directly contributes to the control of insulin secretion. The secretory response of the beta-cell may be directly activated (by *primary stimuli*), modified (by *secondary stimuli*), or inhibited by various agents (see below).

Primary stimuli

Primary stimuli directly affect insulin secretion via a mechanism involving a calcium signal. The transport of calcium through the plasma membrane occurs via several channels, including a specific calcium channel which is sensitive to membrane potential. Calmodulin, a calcium-binding protein, is the major receptor for calcium in the cytoplasm of the beta-cell. The calcium–calmodulin complex activates beta-cell adenylate cyclase, leading to an increase in the net concentration of calcium within the cell. The insulin secretory mechanism is triggered when the calcium concentration reaches a threshold level. Examples of primary stimuli include glucose, amino acids (leucine, arginine, lysine) and fatty acids (short and long chain).

Secondary stimuli

Secondary stimuli modulate the beta-cell secretory response to primary stimuli, but do not directly affect insulin secretion. The mode of action for these agents involves a cyclic AMP signal. Secondary stimuli may increase the response of the beta-cell to primary stimuli by promoting release of calcium from the storage pools and thus increasing the availability of calcium in the cytoplasmic compartment. In the absence of primary stimuli this increase in availability of intracellular calcium does not trigger the insulin secretory mechanism. Examples of secondary stimuli include glucagon (it is for this reason that glucagon is not suitable for treatment of hypoglycaemia in type 2 diabetic patients; see Adverse Effects Focus, p. 37), prostaglandins E_1 and E_2 and sulphonylureas (see pp. 103–106).

Inhibitory agents

Inhibitory agents reduce the response of the beta-cell secretory mechanism to both primary and secondary stimuli. The adrenergic nervous system can inhibit insulin secretion either by releasing the adrenergic neurotransmitter noradrenaline from the nerve terminals in the beta-cell islets or by releasing the hormone adrenaline from the adrenal medulla. Adrenaline and noradrenaline inhibit insulin secretion via the alpha-adrenoceptors on the beta-cell. Activation of the alpha-adreno-ceptors inhibits adenylate cyclase, lowers intracellular cyclic AMP levels, and may also affect the way calcium is handled by the beta-cell. These inhibitory effects may be important during stress when there is a need to elevate blood glucose concentration. An example of an inhibiting agent is diazoxide, which is used for the management of chronic hypo-glycaemia caused by islet cell tumour or hyperplasia, or occasionally for persistent sulphonylurea-induced hypoglycaemia (see pp. 106–107). Diazoxide is not suitable for the management of acute hypoglycaemia induced by exogenous insulin or sulphonylureas (see Adverse Effects Focus, p. 37).

Insulin receptor

The action of insulin is mediated via insulin receptors which are located both on the cell surface of the target tissues and also on intracellular membranes (nucleus, endoplasmic reticulum and Golgi apparatus – may be involved in regulation of protein, DNA and RNA synthesis). The receptor protein consists of four subunits: two extracellular alpha sub-units (linked by disulphide bridges) which bind insulin on the cell surface; and two beta subunits (linked to alpha units by disulphide bridges) which transverse the plasma membrane. The intracellular domain of the beta subunits contains tyrosine-specific protein kinase. It has been proposed that insulin binding to the alpha subunit causes a con-formational change which leads to autophosphorylation of the receptor and activation of tyrosine kinase which in turn initiates the phosphoryl-ation cascade. Insulin–receptor complexes diffuse laterally towards each other within the plane of the plasma membrane and form aggregates. Aggregate-rich areas of the membrane become internalised by the process of endocytosis. The insulin that dissociates from the receptor may then be recycled back to the cell surface. The availability of insulin receptors on the cell surface is controlled by the concentration of extra-cellular insulin. The process of regulating the number of receptors on the cell surface by receptor-mediated endocytosis may be physiologically important for preventing overstimulation of target cells by insulin.

Glucose uptake

Glucose is transported by specific carriers (glucose transporters) which carry glucose across the cell membrane faster than would occur by diffusion alone. A family of six different transporters (GLUT1 to

GLUT6), expressed in different tissues, have been identified. Glucose uptake by muscle (80% of the total body glucose uptake) is mediated by circulating glucose concentrations. The primary form of transporter in skeletal muscle and adipose tissue is GLUT4 (insulin-stimulated glucose transporter). Glucose uptake by the liver, brain, nervous tissue, renal medulla and erythrocytes is independent of glucose concentration.

Insulin preparations have been available for the management of diabetes mellitus for around 75 years. Early porcine and bovine insulin preparations contained other pancreatic proteins (see pp. 97–98) that caused problems such as injection-site lipodystrophy and allergic reactions. These problems have been significantly reduced with better purification methods for bovine and porcine insulins and the development of human-like synthetic insulins (see p. 98).[3]

Pharmacokinetics

Endogenous insulin

Under normal physiological conditions, insulin is secreted from the pancreatic beta-cells into the portal system in response to an increase in blood glucose concentrations above the fasting level (4–5 mmol/L). The pattern of insulin release is bi-phasic, with an initial spike-like first phase followed by a slowly raising second phase. The plasma half-life of insulin is short (approximately 4 min). There is a rapid degradation of the insulin released from the insulin–receptor complex by either soluble (insulin protease) or membrane-bound (insulin glutathione transhydrogenase) enzymes located within the cell (see also Insulin receptor, p. 82). About 50% of the insulin released into the portal system is removed by the liver (which is the major site of insulin degradation), but peripheral tissues also contain specific insulin-degrading enzymes.

Exogenous insulin

Absorption of exogenous insulin into the systemic circulation after subcutaneous injection is variable and influenced by many factors such as: the site, angle and depth of injection; the time of day; the environmental temperature; the phase of the menstrual cycle; and the insulin species and formulation used. Absorption from the arm is faster than from the abdomen and slowest from the thigh (but this is also affected by the type and amount of physical activity). There are no differences in biological potency between human insulin and animal insulin. Human insulin has a faster rate of absorption when administered subcutaneously and a shorter duration of action than animal insulin. The difference between porcine and human insulin is smaller than that between bovine and human insulin. The risk of hypoglycaemia, when switching from bovine to human insulin, may be reduced by a 10% reduction in the daily dose of insulin.[4,5] The rate of insulin absorption may also be affected by smoking (see p. 42), alcohol intake (moderate amounts can cause vaso-dilation of skin blood vessels) and drugs such as propranolol (causing peripheral vasoconstriction) and nifedipine (causing vasodilatation).

In healthy individuals, exogenous insulin has a similar plasma half-life to endogenous insulin of a few minutes and is rapidly metabolised, mainly by the liver. The plasma half-life may be prolonged (up to 13 h) in diabetic patients with high titres of insulin-binding antibodies.

Dosage

Management of type 1 and type 2 diabetes mellitus (by subcutaneous injection)

Starting dose[6,7]

There is no universally accepted, standard, method for calculating the starting dose of insulin in either a newly diagnosed type 1 diabetic patient, or for initiating insulin therapy in a type 2 diabetic patient (when diet and oral antidiabetic therapy have failed). The requirements for insulin vary according to the condition of the individual patient. The requirements are usually high in the presence of concurrent illnesses (e.g. infection) or events (e.g. myocardial infarction, major surgery or injury, puberty, or pregnancy), ketosis or persistent high blood glucose concentrations (see p. 33). Higher doses are also needed in patients who are overweight, in those who do not take regular exercise, or in those who are on concurrent drug therapy which reduces glucose tolerance (see Management Focus, p. 29).

The usual initial dose of insulin in type 1 diabetes ranges from 0.5 to 0.8 units/kg/day depending on the condition and the weight of the patient. For example, in a patient with type 1 diabetes presenting with ketoacidosis or concurrent illness, the requirements for insulin are likely to be initially high (1.0–1.5 units/kg/day). This may increase further as the patient's appetite returns, decrease to around 0.2–0.5 units/kg/day (during the so-called 'honeymoon period' due to production of insulin by the last few beta-cells in the pancreas following recovery from acute ketoacidosis), and then increase again as endogenous insulin production stops. In type 2 diabetes (with insulin resistance) the initial insulin requirements can range from 0.7 to 2.5 units/kg/day. The total daily dose is usually given according to the 'two-thirds rule'; that is, as two-thirds intermediate- or long-acting insulin and one-third as short-acting (soluble) insulin in two divided doses (two-thirds of the total daily dose before breakfast and one-third before the evening meal; see Insulin Dosage Focus, below).

Some diabetes specialists prefer to start off by using a twice-daily injection of an intermediate-acting (e.g. isophane) insulin only and then add a short-acting (e.g. soluble) insulin to cover any hyperglycaemia after breakfast and the evening meal.

Long-term therapy[6–8]

In normal non-diabetic individuals there is a sharp increase in blood insulin concentration in response to an increase in blood glucose following a meal; the concentration then falls and remains at a relatively constant basal level between meals and during the night. The aim of insulin therapy in diabetic patients is to attempt to mimic the physiological process which occurs in the non-diabetic population.

Individual requirements for insulin vary enormously. Long-term insulin therapy must be tailored to suit the individual patient. This can be achieved by using a combination of insulin formulations with varying duration of action (see Table 8.1) and fine-tuning the insulin dosage

INSULIN DOSAGE FOCUS

Calculation of the initial dosage of insulin for a 70-kg man (in hospital) to be given 0.5 units/kg/day

    a. 70 kg × 0.5 units = 35 units per day
    b. 35 rounded up to be divisible by 3 = 36 units per day

Two-thirds of the total daily dose is given in the morning and one-third of the total daily does is given in the evening.

    c. 36 ÷ 3 × 2 = 24 (two-thirds of total daily dose of 36 units)
    d. 36 ÷ 3 × 1 = 12 (one-third of the total daily dose of 36 units)

The dose is made up in the proportion of two-thirds isophane insulin and one-third soluble insulin. Therefore the patient may be given 24 units (as 16 units isophane and 8 units soluble insulin) *before breakfast* and 12 units (as 8 units isophane and 4 units soluble insulin) *before the evening meal.*

N.B. The initial total daily dosage would be lower (50%) if insulin therapy was being initiated while the patient was at home.

Table 8.1 Insulin preparations

Insulin type	Species*	Proprietary names	Product presentation(s)**	Manufacturer
A. QUICK-ACTING				
Action profile† following subcutaneous administration: onset 15 min; time to peak 0.5–1 h; duration 2–5 h				
Insulin aspart	Human	*NovoRapid*	V, C (for *Innovo & Novopen*), D	Novo Nordisk
Insulin lispro	Human	*Humalog*	V, C (for *Autopen*), D	Lilly
B. SHORT-ACTING				
Action profile† following subcutaneous administration: onset 30 min; time to peak 1–3 h; duration 6–8 h				
Soluble insulin	Human (pyr)	*Human Actrapid*	V, C (for *Innovo & Novopen*), D	Novo-Nordisk
	Human (pyr)	*Human Velosulin*	V	Novo-Nordisk
	Human (prb)	*Humulin S*	V, C (for *Autopen*)	Lilly
	Human (prb)	*Humaject S*	D	Lilly
	Human (crb)	*Insuman Rapid*	V, D	Aventis
	Bovine	*Hypurin Bovine Neutral*	V, C (for *Autopen*)	CP Pharm
	Porcine	*Hypurin Porcine Neutral*	V, C (for *Autopen*)	CP Pharm
	Porcine	*Pork Actrapid*	V	Novo-Nordisk
C. INTERMEDIATE-ACTING				
Action profile† following subcutaneous administration: onset 2 h; time to peak 4–12 h; duration up to 24 h				
Isophane insulin	Human (prb)	*Humulin I*	V, C (for *Autopen*), D	Lilly
	Human (crb)	*Insuman Basal*	V, D	Aventis
	Human (pyr)	*Human Insulatard ge*	V, C (for *Autopen, Innovo & Novopen*), D	Novo-Nordisk
	Bovine	*Hypurin Bovine Isophane*	V, C (for *Autopen*)	CP Pharm
	Porcine	*Hypurin Porcine Isophane*	V, C (for *Autopen*)	CP Pharm
	Porcine	*Pork Insulatard*	V	Novo-Nordisk

D. MIXED INSULINS

Action profile† following subcutaneous administration: onset up to 2 h; time to peak 4–12 h; duration up to 24 h

Biphasic insulin aspart	Human	Novomix 30	C (for Innovo & Novopen), D	Novo-Nordisk
Biphasic insulin lispro	Human	Humalog Mix 25, 50	C (for Autopen), D	Lilly
Biphasic isophane insulin	Human (pyr)	Human Mixtard 30 ge	V	Novo-Nordisk
	Human (pyr)	Human Mixtard 10, 20, 30, 40, 50	C (for Autopen, Innovo & Novopen), D	Novo-Nordisk
	Human (prb)	Humulin M2, M3, M5	V, C (for Autopen), D	Lilly
	Human (crb)	Insuman Comb 15, 25, 50	V, D	Aventis
	Porcine	Hypurin Porcine 30/70 mix	V, C (for Autopen)	CP Pharm
	Porcine	Pork Mixtard 30	V	Novo-Nordisk

E. LONG-ACTING

Action profile† following subcutaneous administration: Onset 2–4 h; Time to peak 6–20 h; Duration up to 36 h

Insulin zinc suspension (mixed)	Human (pyr)	Human Monotard	V	Novo-Nordisk
	Human (prb)	Humulin Lente	V	Novo-Nordisk
	Bovine	Hypurin Bovine Lente	V	CP Pharm
Insulin zinc suspension (crystalline)	Human (prb)	Humulin Zn	V	Lilly
	Human (pyr)	Human Ultratard	V	Novo-Nordisk
Protamine zinc insulin	Bovine	Hypurin Bovine Protamine Zinc	V	CP Pharm

F. LONG-ACTING ANALOGUE

Insulin glargine	Human	Lantus	V, D	Aventis

* Species: aspart (insulin amino acid proline at B28 replaced with aspartic acid) lispro (insulin amino acid sequence B28-B29 reversed to lysine-proline); glargine (insulin amino acid asparagine at A21 replaced with glycine and two arginine residues added B31 and B32); crb (chain recombinant bacterial); emp (enzymatically modified porcine); ge (genetic engineering); prb (proinsulin recombinant bacterial); pyr (precursor yeast recombinant).

** C, Cartridges (1.5 and/or 3 mL) for injection devices; D, prefilled (3 mL) disposable injection devices; V, vials (10 mL).

In UK all insulin preparations are prescription-only medicines (PoM) and available-only as 100 units/mL.

† Action profiles are affected by the dose, injection site, injection technique, exercise, temperature and insulin species.

according to the patient's individual blood glucose profile (see Adjustment of insulin dosage based on blood glucose concentrations, p. 91).

It is important for patients to be aware of their individual blood glucose targets and treatment goals (see Glycaemic Control Focus, p. 48). For example, a young person with diabetes can aim to keep their blood glucose level between 5 and 7 mmol/L, whereas for an elderly person living alone the risk of hypoglycaemia is higher, and therefore a safer target would be to aim for blood glucose levels of between 6 and 10 mmol/L. An awareness of the patient's eating habits is also important. Administration of two-thirds of the total daily dose of insulin before breakfast assumes that the patient will consume two-thirds of the total daily calories at breakfast and lunch. This may not necessarily be applicable to all patients.[7]

Insulin regimens

In non-diabetic individuals, there is a sharp rise in insulin after consumption of a meal that is superimposed on a constant basal level of insulin secretion. Insulin dosage regimens attempt to mimic this pattern by using combinations of quick- or short-acting insulins, which match the rise in insulin after meals, and intermediate- or long-acting insulins, which provide the basal level of insulin (to prevent fasting hyperglycaemia). This is sometimes referred to as the 'basal-bolus' regimen. Ideal glycaemic control is often difficult to achieve, as there is a delay in achieving peak plasma insulin levels after subcutaneous injection. There is also a problem in providing a constant background level of insulin. Under normal physiological conditions basal insulin levels are constant, whereas with injected insulin, absorption into the circulation is variable (see pp. 83–84) with peaks and troughs in insulin levels. It is therefore necessary to determine insulin dosage and regimen on an individual basis by using blood glucose monitoring (see p. 45), with special attention to diet (see Chapter 6) and exercise (see pp. 39–41).

There are three general types of insulin regimens:

- Twice-daily injection regimen – mixture of an intermediate-acting insulin and a short-acting insulin twice daily (before breakfast and evening meal).
- Multiple injection regimen – short-acting insulin before each meal and intermediate-acting insulin or long-acting insulin at bedtime.
- Once-daily injection regimen – long-acting insulin in the morning with or without short-acting insulin.

Twice-daily injection regimen   This regimen assumes that the patient is consuming three main meals and three snacks during the day at regular times. The day is divided into four parts, with the hyperglycaemia following breakfast and evening meal being covered by the short-acting component of the insulin dosage (i.e. periods immediately after injection) and any hyperglycaemia during the afternoon and night being covered by the intermediate-acting component of the insulin dosage. The patient usually starts by injecting two-thirds of the total daily dosage of insulin in the morning and one-third in the evening (see Insulin Dosage Focus, p. 85). The patient can then adjust the division of the daily dosage and the ratio of short-acting/intermediate-acting insulin according to their individual blood glucose concentration profile during the day based on blood glucose monitoring results.

The twice-daily regimen offers the convenience of fitting in well with the standard working day, and the patient does not have to take insulin at work. However, the profiles of blood glucose and insulin concentrations achieved during the day differ significantly from normal physiological profiles. There are no sharp increases in insulin levels after meals, as the absorption of insulin after subcutaneous administration is slow in comparison to the rise in blood glucose levels. This means that the patient is hyperglycaemic for about an hour after the consumption of each meal. The profile of insulin concentrations between meals and during the night also differs significantly from the basal levels of endogenous insulin present under normal physiological conditions. Following the injection of insulin before an evening meal, the concentrations of insulin are higher than required during the evening and then gradually fall during the night. This means that most patients require an evening snack before bedtime in order to avoid nocturnal hypoglycaemia (see Adverse Effects Focus, p. 37).

The components of short-acting (soluble) insulin and intermediate-acting (isophane) insulin have been prescribed as separate preparations in the past. This provided flexibility in allowing adjustments in the ratio of the two components of insulin when fine-tuning the dosage. However, the complication of the patient having to draw up different quantities of two different insulins and mix them in a syringe before injecting the dose caused problems such as reduced accuracy of the dose (e.g. interchanging the amount of the two types of insulin by mistake) and contamination of the short-acting (soluble) insulin with intermediate-acting (isophane) insulin (affecting the time of onset and duration of action of the short-acting insulin). Pre-mixed insulins that contain fixed ratios of short-acting (soluble) and intermediate-acting (isophane) insulins allow less flexibility in fine-tuning the dosage, but are much simpler and more convenient to use, particularly when injected by using insulin pen devices (see Table 8.1).

Multiple injection regimen   With this regimen, the short-acting insulin controls the hyperglycaemia that occurs after each meal, and the intermediate or long-acting insulin provides the background 'basal' level of insulin required during the night to control fasting hyperglycaemia. Half of the total daily requirement is given as short-acting (e.g. soluble) insulin, and half as either intermediate (e.g. isophane) or less commonly long-acting insulin (e.g. insulin zinc suspension (mixed), sometimes referred to as 'lente'). Insulin lispro is now increasingly being used instead of soluble insulin as the short-acting component of this regimen. It has the advantage of being absorbed more rapidly than soluble insulin (see p. 100).

This regimen allows the patient flexibility of varying the timing and content of their meals and also allows them to omit the daytime snacks (though the bedtime snack should never be omitted because of the risk of nocturnal hypoglycaemia). The patient can make appropriate adjustments to the short-acting insulin dosage according to the level of activity and the size and content of the meals. Insulin pen devices provide a safe and convenient method for carrying and injecting insulin during the day. This regimen is suitable for adolescents and some children who do not like adhering to a strict predetermined daily routine. However, the regimen relies on frequent finger-prick blood glucose measurements for optimal control. Some adolescents with type 1 diabetes may deliberately skip doses and meals because it does not fit into their day, and thus they are at increased risk of diabetic ketoacidosis (see pp. 33–34).

The appropriateness of the multiple injection regimen must be considered on an individual basis. Intensive insulin therapy is not appropriate in children under 7 years (who are at risk of brain damage from hypoglycaemia) and patients with severe diabetic complications (there is no evidence that tight glycaemic control reverses established microvascular complications). Caution is also advised in patients with established coronary or cerebrovascular disease, as rapidly lowering the blood glucose levels can cause significant changes in cardiac output, heart rate, blood pressure and cerebral blood flow that can lead to acute vascular problems.

A slightly less flexible variation of the multiple injection regimen is injection of long-acting and short-acting insulin in the morning, and short-acting insulin in the evening. With this regimen, the peak effect of the long-acting insulin occurs during the day and may provide reasonable glycaemic control during the day with fewer injections.

Once-daily injection regimen This regimen rarely achieves normal blood glucose levels during the day, but provides sufficient background insulin over 24 h to prevent severe hyperglycaemia and hence reduces the risks of diabetic emergencies. It may be useful for patients in whom the evening blood glucose concentrations are not high enough to make a second dose of short-acting insulin absolutely necessary, or for elderly patients preferring single daily injections or for those having to rely on others (e.g. community nurses) to administer the insulin. However, the greater risk of hypoglycaemia and the nutritional status in the elderly should be borne in mind when long-acting insulin is administered.

Adjustment of insulin dosage based on blood glucose concentrations[2]

The dosage of insulin can be fine-tuned by patients according to their individual needs by basing adjustments on their blood or urine glucose profiles (see Insulin Dosage Focus, p. 92). The aim is for the patient to achieve the best possible glycaemic control without becoming obsessive about glucose monitoring and insulin dosage. The emphasis should be on the profiles of blood glucose concentrations throughout the day over several days. Adjustment of insulin doses is usually only necessary if the blood glucose concentrations are consistently too low or too high over a period of about 3 days unless the patient is showing signs of ketoacidosis or experiencing symptoms of hypoglycaemia, in which case it is advisable for the patient to seek medical help (see p. 37). Patients should be advised not to alter their insulin dosage by more than 4 units at any one time.

Changing type of insulin used or insulin regimen

The range and types of insulins available has increased over the past few years. This means that a wide range of insulin regimens are possible to meet the needs of the individual person with diabetes. The main aim for changing the type of insulin or regimen used should be to improve both the short-term and long-term quality of life; for example, to reduce risk of hypoglycaemia or hyperglycaemia, to simplify daily routine or to suit a particular lifestyle or life change (pregnancy, physical illness, shiftwork, new exercise regimen). Appropriate education is the key element for any

INSULIN DOSAGE FOCUS

Adjustment of insulin dosage according to blood glucose concentration profiles

---

A patient on a twice-daily injection regimen (see p. 89) has too many fluctuations in blood glucose concentrations which fall outside their goal of maintaining blood glucose within 5–10 mmol/L. With regimen A, the day is divided into four divisions with the option of altering either the morning or the evening dose of insulin and also the option of altering the short-acting or the intermediate-acting component of each dose. The decision as to which dose requires alteration depends on the time(s) during the day at which the blood glucose concentrations fluctuate outside the desired range. In general, an adjustment of the morning dose is likely to be needed if the blood glucose concentration is too low or too high before lunch (short-acting component of the dose) or before the evening meal (intermediate-acting component of the dose). An adjustment of the evening dose may be necessary if the blood glucose concentration is too low or too high before breakfast (intermediate-acting component of the dose) or before bedtime (short-acting component of the dose). However, caution is advised when considering an increase in the evening dose because of the risk of nocturnal hypoglycaemia. High blood glucose concentrations before breakfast may be due to rebound hyperglycaemia (sometimes referred to as the *Somogyi effect*) which can result from nocturnal hypoglycaemia. It is important to check for any symptoms of nocturnal hypoglycaemia such as disturbed dreams or copious sweating, although some patients do not experience such symptoms. The blood glucose concentration before bedtime should not be lower than 6.0 mmol/L (see Adverse Effects Focus, p. 37).

---

change to lead to a successful outcome. Any change in insulin therapy is a major change for the individual concerned as it can alter glycaemic control, incidence of hypoglycaemia and general well-being.

Adverse effects

Hypoglycaemia

Hypoglycaemia is a major cause of anxiety in patients and their relatives, and is the most common complication of insulin therapy. The risk of hypoglycaemia is highest before meals and at night. Causes include irregular eating habits, unusual level of exercise or excessive alcohol intake (see Adverse Effects Focus, p. 38). A variation in the rate of absorption of insulin from the injection site may also precipitate hypoglycaemia. Nocturnal hypoglycaemia can be caused by a high evening insulin dose. The onset of hypoglycaemia can be sudden and without warning in long-term diabetic patients. Loss of hypoglycaemic awareness can be a serious hazard, especially if a hypoglycaemic episode occurs while the patient is driving or operating machinery. Some patients have reported loss of hypoglycaemic awareness following the change from animal to human insulin. It has been suggested that this may be due to species differences in the effect of insulin on the central nervous system, but clinical evidence for a difference in hypoglycaemic episodes between human and animal insulins is lacking. A review carried out by the Nuffield Institute for Health concluded that human insulin does not increase the frequency or affect the symptoms of hypoglycaemia among the general population of people with diabetes.[9] The results showed it was unlikely that human insulin affected hypoglycaemia, but it is impossible to prove that human insulin does not cause problems. Animal insulins remain available for patients who want them (see Table 8.1).

Lipodystrophy

Early porcine and bovine insulin preparations contained other pancreatic proteins which caused injection-site lipodystrophy and both local and systemic allergic reactions. These problems have been significantly reduced with better purification methods for bovine and porcine insulins and the development of human-like synthetic insulins (see p. 97).[3]

Cardiovascular effects

There has been some concern that insulin therapy in type 2 diabetic patients may cause or exacerbate underlying cardiovascular disease due to insulin resistance and hyperinsulinaemia (see Chapter 7). The association between hyperinsulinaemia and cardiovascular disease is based on epidemiological data from people with hyperinsulinaemia who were not diabetic.[10] There is no evidence to support the hypothesis that insulin treatment in type 2 diabetes increases the risk of myocardial infarction even though the fasting insulin concentrations are higher in those treated with insulin compared to other treatment groups.[11]

Weight gain

Insulin therapy is associated with weight gain, which is considered undesirable in obese type 2 diabetic patients as it may increase insulin resistance. Weight gain in type 2 diabetic patients may be due to overeating as a result of inappropriate insulin dosage, or to the time of administration which can lead to symptoms of hypoglycaemia and feeling of hunger (see pp. 35–38).

Drug interactions

Hypoglycaemic effect enhanced

Drugs that increase insulin sensitivity and glucose utilisation and decrease hepatic glucose output (HGO) can cause hypoglycaemia in type 1 and type 2 diabetic patients treated with insulin. Drugs that stimulate endogenous insulin release can cause hypoglycaemia in type 2 diabetic patients treated with insulin or sulphonylureas.[12–14]

Alcohol

For a discussion on alcohol and hypoglycaemia, see p. 42.

Angiotensin-converting enzyme (ACE) inhibitors

ACE inhibitors may increase insulin sensitivity in diabetic patients. The mechanism is not fully understood, though it has been suggested that ACE inhibitors increase insulin sensitivity and glucose utilisation, whilst an alteration in kidney function may also be a contributory factor.

Severe hypoglycaemic episodes have been reported with ACE inhibitors (captopril, enalapril and lisinopril) in type 2 diabetic patients being treated with insulin and sulphonylureas. A 3.5-fold increase in risk of developing hypoglycaemia associated with ACE inhibitor therapy has been reported.[15,16] Diabetic control should be monitored closely, particularly when initiating ACE inhibitor therapy. The patient should be warned of the possibility of an unpredictable hypoglycaemic episode. It may be necessary, in some cases, to reduce the dose of antidiabetic therapy.

Anabolic steroids

Nandrolone, methandienone, testosterone and stanozolol enhance the action of insulin. The dosage of insulin may need to be reduced.

Beta-blockers

The adrenergic nervous system is involved in the counter-regulatory responses to insulin-induced lowering of blood glucose. Under normal physiological conditions, adrenaline increases heart rate and hepatic glucose output in response to a fall in blood glucose levels. Non-selective beta-blockers such as propranolol affect $beta_2$-adrenoceptors in the heart, peripheral vasculature, bronchi, pancreas and the liver. A decrease in hypoglycaemic awareness is due to inhibition of the early 'adrenergic' warning signs of hypoglycaemia such as tremor and palpitations (but not hunger and sweating). Inhibition of hepatic glucose output causes a delay in the recovery from hypoglycaemia. There also may be an increase in blood pressure due to vasoconstriction caused by unopposed effects of adrenaline on alpha-adrenoceptors. Vasoconstriction may also aggravate poor peripheral circulation in some diabetic patients. 'Cardioselective' beta-blockers mainly affect the $beta_1$-adrenoceptors in the heart, whereas non-selective beta-blockers also significantly affect $beta_2$-receptors in other organs. Therefore cardioselective beta-blockers may be preferable if beta-blocker therapy is necessary for a diabetic patient (see Adverse Effects Focus, below, and Management Focus, pp. 23–25). Some beta-blockers have the capacity to stimulate as well as block adrenoceptors – an effect that is usually referred to as intrinsic sympathomimetic activity (ISA) or partial agonist activity. Acebutolol and oxprenolol have partial agonist activity for $beta_1$-adrenoceptors, whereas pindolol and celiprolol have partial agonist activity for $beta_2$-adrenoceptors.

Severe hypoglycaemia (with coma in some cases) has been reported with propranolol, pindolol and timolol eye-drops in patients on insulin. Associated marked increases in blood pressure have also been reported with propranolol and metoprolol. Non-selective beta-blockers should be

ADVERSE EFFECTS FOCUS

Adrenoceptor selectivity of beta-blockers	
Selectivity	**Beta-blockers**
A. Cardioselective	
$Beta_1$	Atenolol, Betaxolol, Bisoprolol, Metoprolol, Acebutolol, Esmolol
B. Non-selective	
$Beta_1$ and $Beta_2$	Carvedilol, Nadolol, Oxprenolol, Pindolol, Propranolol, Sotalol, Timolol
$Beta_1$ and $Alpha_2$	Celiprolol
$Beta_1$, $Beta_2$ and $Alpha_1$	Labetolol

avoided (see Adverse Effects Focus, p. 95). Beta-blocker use in a diabetic patient should be closely monitored. The patient should be warned that some of the early warning signs of hypoglycaemia may not occur.

Disopyramide

Severe hypoglycaemia has been reported. The mechanism is not understood, but insulin secretion may be affected. Patients should be closely monitored.

Fluoxetine

This enhances the effects of insulin by increasing insulin sensitivity. Patients should be closely monitored.

Mebendazole

An improvement in glycaemic control in diabetic patients on initiation of mebendazole therapy has been reported. This effect may be due to an enhancement in insulin secretion by mebendazole.[17]

Monoamine oxidase inhibitors (MAOIs)

The hypoglycaemic effect possibly occurs via direct action on the pancreas with insulin release. This is an established interaction, but the mechanism is not fully understood. It may be necessary to reduce the dose of hypoglycaemic drug if MAOIs are used concomitantly. Moclobemide, a reversible inhibitor of monoamine oxidase type A (RIMA), does not have this effect.

Quinine and quinidine

Hypoglycaemia has been reported in non-diabetic patients treated with quinine or quinidine for falciparum malaria or leg cramps. The mechanism involves direct stimulation of the pancreas, causing insulin release. It may be prudent to monitor diabetic control closely when using these compounds concomitantly with antidiabetic therapy.

Salicylates

Aspirin and other salicylates can lower blood glucose levels. The effect of salicylates on glucose tolerance is complex. High doses can cause hypoglycaemia as well as hyperglycaemia. The suggested mechanism is that salicylates cause hypoglycaemia by increasing glucose utilisation and inhibiting glucose synthesis from alanine. Hypoglycaemia does not appear to be a problem with small analgesic doses of aspirin.

Tetracyclines

There have been few reports of the effects of insulin and sulphonylureas being increased by oxytetracycline and doxycycline. The mechanism is not fully understood. It may be necessary to reduce the dose of hypo-glycaemic drug with concomitant use.

Drugs impairing glucose tolerance

See Management Focus, p. 29.

Preparations

See Table 8.1.

Insulin sources

The four sources of insulin for pharmaceutical use[18] are:

- Conventional insulins.
- Highly purified insulins.
- Semisynthetic human insulin (modified porcine).
- Biosynthetic human insulin.

Conventional insulins

These early insulin preparations were obtained by extraction from bovine or porcine pancreases and purified by recrystallisation only. These preparations also contained proinsulin, insulin derivatives (esters, arginine insulin, desamidoinsulin) and other pancreatic peptides (glucagon, pancreatic polypeptide, somatostatin, vasoactive intestinal peptide).

Highly purified insulins

These insulin preparations are purified by improved purification methods. The method of purification is sometimes indicated by initials which form part of the name of the preparation, for example:

- *SP (single peak)*: insulin purified by crystallisation and gel filtration. This method of purification reduces the content of proinsulin but does not affect content of insulin derivatives and other pancreatic peptides.
- *MC (monocomponent), SC (single component), RI (rarely immunogenic)*: insulin purified by gel filtration and ion-exchange chromatography. This method further reduces the proinsulin content and also reduces the content of insulin derivatives and other pancreatic peptides.

Semisynthetic human insulin (modified porcine)

Human insulin differs structurally from porcine insulin by one amino acid (position 30 on the B chain) and from bovine insulin by three amino acids (position 30 on the B chain and two amino acids on the A chain). The letters *emp* stand for enzymatically modified porcine.

Biosynthetic human insulin

These are human insulins produced by recombinant DNA technology. The method of production is usually indicated by a suffix of initials:

- *ge*: genetic engineering. This form is made from a genetically engineered strain of bacterium, usually *E. coli*.
- *crb*: chain recombinant bacterial. Human insulin chains are produced by inserting recombinant DNA into a bacterium followed by chemical synthesis to the human insulin molecule.
- *prb*: proinsulin recombinant bacterial. Proinsulin is produced by inserting the proinsulin gene into a bacterium and then cleaved to the human insulin molecule.
- *pyr*: precursor yeast recombinant. Proinsulin is produced by inserting the proinsulin gene into yeast cells and then cleaved to the human insulin molecule.

Insulin formulations

The rate of absorption of insulin after subcutaneous administration can be modified by the formulation of the preparation. Short-acting formulations are used for the management of post-prandial hyperglycaemia. Long-acting (modified release) formulations were developed to provide background 'basal' insulin levels.

Short-acting insulin

Soluble insulin (insulin injection, neutral insulin, regular insulin, unmodified insulin) This preparation has not been formulated to modify the duration of action of insulin. Insulin molecules exist as hexamers in solution which disassociate into dimers and monomers after subcutaneous injection and before absorption. When administered subcutaneously, the time for onset of action is about 30 min, with peak effect occurring after 2–4 h. The effect lasts for 6–8 h. Soluble insulin needs to be injected approximately 30 min before a meal. The low initial bioavailability of insulin with this preparation has been associated with early post-prandial hyperglycaemia. Its duration of action has been associated with inappropriate hyperinsulinaemia, and increased risk of hypoglycaemia.

Long-acting (modified release) formulations

Protamine zinc insulin (protamine 'retard' insulin) Protamine zinc insulin contains insulin, zinc chloride and excess amounts of protamine (molecular). Insulin is released slowly from an insulin–zinc–protamine complex.

Isophane insulin (isophane protamine insulin, NPH) Isophane insulin contains equal amounts (molecular) of insulin and protamine. Insulin is released slowly from an insulin–protamine complex.

Insulin zinc suspensions (IZS) IZS consist of insulin combined with zinc to form complexes or crystals from which insulin is released slowly. There are three types:

- *Insulin zinc suspension (amorphous) (semilente).* Insulin combined with zinc ions to form complexes. Preparation contains particles with variable shapes (<2 mμ). Onset: approximately 2 h, peak: 4–12 h, duration: up to 24 h.
- *Insulin zinc suspension (mixed) (insulin lente).* Insulin combined with zinc ions to form complexes. Preparation contains a mixture of particles (rhombohedral crystals, 10–40 mμ plus particles with variable shapes, <2 mμ). Onset: 2–4 h, peak: 4–12 h, duration: up to 24 h.
- *Insulin zinc suspension (crystalline) (ultralente).* Insulin crystallised with zinc into insoluble particles (rhombohedral crystals, 10–40 mμ). Onset: 3–4 h, peak: 14–20 h, duration: 24–36 h.

Mixed insulin preparations   Isophane and soluble insulins can be mixed within the same syringe shortly before injection. This does not appear to modify the action of either insulin, and premixed insulins are now available. These preparations provide fixed ratios of soluble insulin and isophane insulin (see Table 8.1), which reduces patient error in measuring different doses of different insulins. However, the flexibility for dosage adjustment is also reduced. It is not possible to mix soluble insulin and zinc insulins in this way as soluble insulin forms complexes with free zinc ions, and this effectively prolongs its duration of action.

Insulin analogues

Rapid-acting insulin analogues

Insulin lispro (short-acting insulin analogue, recombinant human insulin analogue)   Insulin lispro is an insulin analogue produced by changing the sequence of amino acids 28 (proline) and 29 (lysine) on chain B of the insulin molecule to amino acids 28 (lysine) and 29 (proline), respectively (see Figure 8.1, p. 80). This analogue displays different physical properties to soluble insulin (human, porcine or bovine). Insulin lispro exists as a monomer in solution and does not have a tendency to self-associate. After subcutaneous administration, insulin lispro has a more rapid onset of action (approximately 15 min) and a shorter duration of effect (2–5 h) than soluble insulin. It can be injected just before meals. The rapid onset of action combined with shorter duration of effect of insulin lispro provides better post-prandial glycaemic control.[19] Insulin lispro has been complexed with protamine to produce an intermediate-acting form, which is available as a biphasic preparation

Insulin aspart (short-acting insulin analogue, recombinant human insulin analogue)   Insulin aspart is an insulin analogue produced by changing amino acid 28 (proline) on chain B of the insulin molecule to aspartic acid (see Figure 8.1, p. 80). It has a more rapid onset and shorter duration of action than soluble insulin. It may be injected immediately before a meal rather than 30 min before a meal, as required with soluble insulin. The shorter duration of action may reduce the risk of hypoglycaemia.[20]

Long-acting insulin analogues

Insulin glargine (basal insulin analogue, recombinant human insulin analogue)   Insulin glargine is an insulin analogue produced by changing amino acid 21 (asparagine) on chain A of the insulin molecule to glycine and by adding two arginine residues 31 and 32 to chain B (see Figure 8.1, p. 80). These changes to the human insulin molecule enhances the formation of hexamers and increases solubility in an acidic environment. Insulin glargine precipitates in the neutral pH environment of human subcutaneous tissue and hence has a prolonged absorption time. Zinc has been added to some formulations of insulin glargine to further extend the absorption time.[21]

References

1. Montague, W. *Diabetes and the Endocrine Pancreas, A Biochemical Approach*. London: Croom Helm, 1983.
2. Ido Y, Vindigni A, Chang K, *et al*. Prevention of vascular and neural dysfunction in diabetic rats by C-peptide. *Science* 1997; 277: 563–566.
3. Hoffman A, Ziv E. Pharmacokinetic considerations of new insulin formulations and routes of administration. *Clin Pharmacokinet* 1997; 33: 285–301.
4. Everett J, Kerr D. Changing from porcine to human insulin. *Drugs* 1994; 47:286–296.
5. Anonymous. Insulin preparations – time to rationalise. *Drug Ther Bull* 1996; 34: 11–14.
6. Grahame-Smith D G, Aronson J K (eds). *Oxford Textbook of Clinical Pharmacology and Drug Therapy*, 2nd edition. New York: Oxford University Press, 1992: 378–391.
7. Koda-Kimble M A, Young L Y (eds). *Applied Therapeutics: The Clinical Use of Drugs*, 5th edition. Vancouver: Applied Therapeutics Inc., 1992: Chapter 72.
8. McDowell J R S, Gordon D (eds). *Diabetes: Caring for Patients in the Community*. London: Churchill Livingstone, 1996.
9. Williams R, Airey M, Bennett C, *et al*. *Human and Animal Insulins Compared. A Report Commissioned by the British Diabetic Association*. Division of Public Health, Nuffield Institute for Health, University of Leeds. 4 July 2000.
10. Turner R C, Holman R R. Insulin use in NIDDM. Rationale based on pathophysiology of disease. *Diabetes Care* 1990; 13: 1011–1019.
11. UK Prospective Diabetes Study (UKPDS) Group. Intensive blood-glucose control with sulphonylureas or insulin compared with conventional treatment and risk of complications in patients with type 2 diabetes (UKPDS 33). *Lancet* 1998; 352: 837–853.
12. Stockley I H. *Drug Interactions*, 4th edition. London: Pharmaceutical Press, 1996.
13. Scheen A J, Lefebvre P J. Antihyperglycaemic agents. Drug interactions of clinical importance. *Drug Safety* 1995; 12: 32–45.
14. Ferner R E. Drug-induced hypoglycaemia. *Adverse Drug Reaction Bulletin* 1996; No. 179: 679–682.
15. Anonymous. Tayside DARTS database review of prescribing and hospitalisation data for diabetic patients. *Pharm J* 1996; 257: 483.

16. Morris A D, Boyle D I R, McMahon A D, *et al.* ACE inhibitor use is associated with hospitalization for severe hypoglycaemia in patients with diabetes. *Diabetes Care* 1997; 20: 1363–1367.

17. O'Byrne S, Feely J. Effects of drugs on glucose tolerance in non-insulin-dependent diabetics (Part II). *Drugs* 1990; 40: 203–219.

18. Sweetman, S (ed.). *Martindale: the Complete Drug Reference*, 33rd edition. London: Pharmaceutical Press, 2002.

19. Anonymous. Humalog – a new insulin analogue. *Drug Ther Bull* 1997; 35: 57–58.

20. Simpson KL, Spencer CM. Insulin aspart. *Drugs* 1999; 57: 759–765.

21. Gillies P S, Figgitt D P, Lamb H M. Insulin glargine. *Drugs* 2000; 59: 253–260.

9

Sulphonylureas

Indications

Sulphonylureas (Figure 9.1) are used for the management of type 2 diabetes when dietary management alone has failed. Sulphonylureas may be used use as monotherapy or in combination with metformin or insulin (see Chapter 7).

Mechanism of action

The potential usefulness of sulphonylureas in diabetes was discovered by accident in the 1940s when severe hypoglycaemia was observed in patients with typhoid fever who were being treated with a thiodiazole derivative of sulphonamide.[1] This led to the development of carbutamide. Carbutamide and another sulphonylurea compound, methexamide, were subsequently withdrawn from clinical use because of their toxic side effects. However, closely related compounds such as chlorpropamide and tolbutamide, the so-called 'first-generation sulphonylureas', are still in clinical use (see Table 9.1). The relatively more recent 'second-generation sulphonylureas' such as glibenclamide and gliclazide display a higher potency than the first-generation compounds. The elimination half-life of a sulphonylurea does not give a true indication of the duration of hypoglycaemic action, as this is also dependent upon the presence of any active metabolites. Therefore the duration of hypoglycaemic action of the individual sulphonylurea (rather than the distinction according to potency or the chronological classification) is the significant factor when choosing a sulphonylurea for clinical use. Sulphonylureas stimulate insulin secretion by acting as a secondary stimulus on pancreatic beta-cells (see Insulin secretion, p. 80). The antidiabetic action of sulphonylureas is mediated via specific receptors on beta-cells. The interaction of sulphonylureas with these receptors results in the closure of potassium channels in the membrane leading to depolarisation and an influx of calcium, which in turn triggers insulin release from the beta-cell secretory granules. Glimepiride, a new

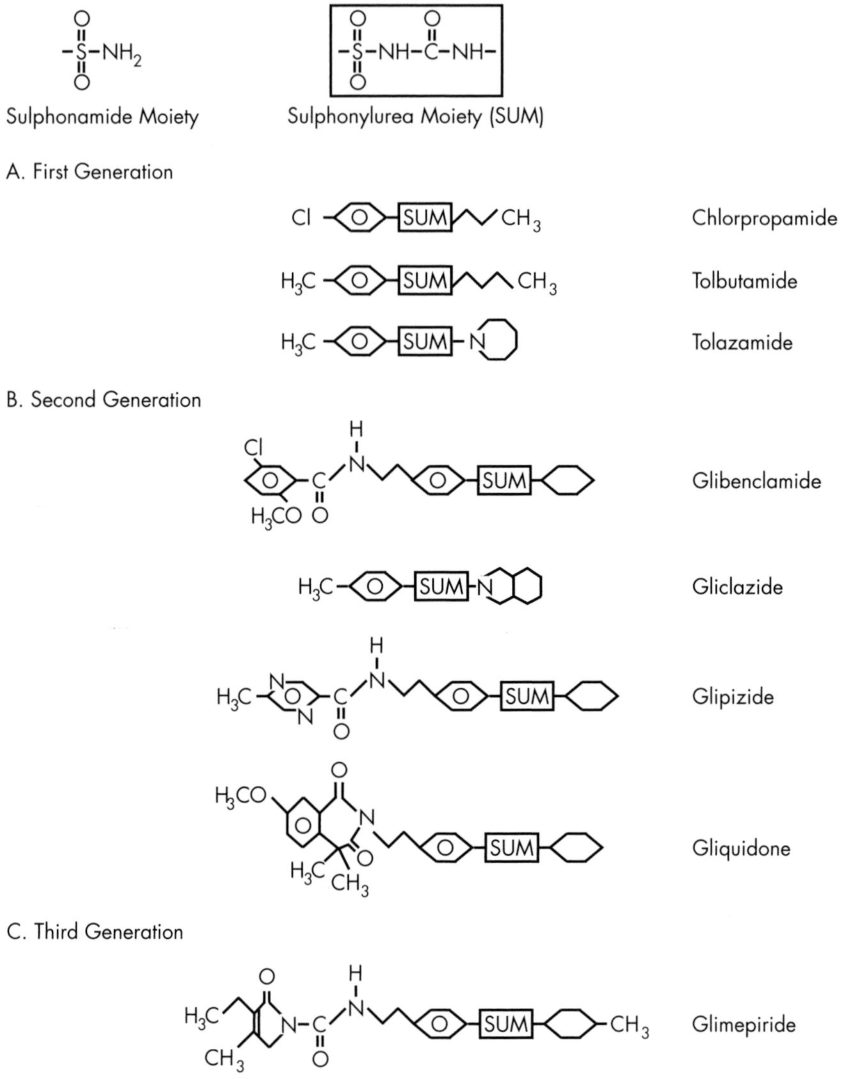

Figure 9.1   Sulphonylureas.

sulphonylurea, binds to a different protein of the sulphonylurea receptor from that of the other sulphonylureas but has the same effect on the
insulin secretory mechanism. It is still a matter of debate as to whether
the action of sulphonylureas is confined to the islet beta-cells in the

Table 9.1 Oral antidiabetic drugs

Antidiabetic drugs	Half-life t1/2 (h)	Duration of effect (h)	Daily dose	Tablet strength (mg)	Comments	Proprietary name(s) (UK)	Manufacturer(s) (UK)
A. SULPHONYLUREAS							
First generation (low potency)							
Chlorpropamide	24–48	24–72	250 mg (elderly 100 mg); max. 500 mg	100 & 250	Very long-acting, can cause severe hypoglycaemia and unpleasant facial flushing in susceptible individuals		Sussex
Tolbutamide	3–28	6–10	0.5–1.5 g; max. 2 g	500	Absorption affected by food		Alpharma, APS, Hillcross
Second generation (high potency)							
Glibenclamide	2–4 may be longer	20–29	5 mg (elderly 2.5 mg); max. 15 mg	2.5 & 5	Elimination half-life may be longer. Bioavailability variation between micronised and non-micronised formulations. Absorption affected by food	*Daonil, Semi-Daonil, Diabetamide, Euglucon*	APS, Ashbourne, Aventis, CP Pharm, Generics, Hillcross, Hoechst Marion Roussel
Gliclazide	6–15	10–15	40–80 mg; max. 160 mg (single dose); max. 320 mg (divided doses)	80		*Diamicron*	Alpharma, APS, Dominion, Generics, Hillcross, Servier
Glipizide	1–5	14–16	2.5–5 mg; max. 15 mg (single dose); max. 40 mg (divided doses)	2.5 & 5	Absorption delayed by food and hyperglycaemia	*Glibenese, Minodiab*	Alpharma, Hillcross, Pfizer, Pharmacia
Gliquidone			15 mg; max. 60 mg (single dose); max. 180 mg (divided doses)	30		*Glurenorm*	Sanofi-Synthelabo
Third generation (high potency – different binding site on sulphonylurea 'receptor')							
Glimepiride	5–8		1–4 mg; max. 6 mg	1, 2, 3, & 4		*Amaryl*	Hoechst Marion Roussel
B. BIGUANIDES							
Metformin	3		1.5–1.7 g; max. 3 g (preferable limit 2 g)	500 & 800	Gastrointestinal disturbances may persist at higher doses	*Glucophage*	Alpharma, APS, CP Pharm, Generics
C. ALPHA GLUCOSIDASE INHIBITORS							
Acarbose	Negligible absorption		50–300 mg; max. 600 mg	50 & 100	Increase dose over 6–8 weeks to reduce side-effects	*Glucobay*	Bayer
D. THIAZOLIDINEDIONES (PPAR-γ-agonists)							
Pioglitazone	7	24	15–30 mg	15, 30	For combined therapy only	*Actos*	Takeda
Rosiglitazone	3–4		4–8 mg	4, 8	For combined therapy only. Increase dose after 8 weeks	*Avandia*	Glaxo Smith Kline
E. MEGLITINIDES							
Nateglinide	1.5		180 mg in divided doses; max 540 mg	60, 120, 180	To be taken within 30 min before meal	*Starlix*	Novartis
Repaglinide	1		0.5–4 mg single dose; max 16 mg daily	0.5, 1, 2	To be taken within 30 min before meal. Adjust dose at 1–2 weekly intervals	*NovoNorm*	Novo Nordisk

pancreas or whether extrapancreatic sites are also involved. It has been suggested that sulphonylureas reduce insulin resistance via an extra-pancreatic mechanism by increasing the number of insulin receptors (see p. 82) on target cell membranes (with enhancement of post-receptor pathways of glucose metabolism) and also by altering the hepatic extraction of insulin. The existence of any extrapancreatic action of sulphonylureas is controversial.[2]

Pharmacokinetics

Sulphonylureas are extensively bound to plasma proteins. They are metabolised in the liver and produce metabolites (active and inactive) that are excreted mainly in the urine. There are differences in the rate of absorption, metabolism and excretion between different sulphonylureas. Bioavailability is affected by the time of ingestion in relation to food and blood glucose levels. A reduction in plasma glipizide levels with increasing hyperglycaemia in type 2 diabetic patients has been reported. It is likely that hyperglycaemia affects absorption of all sulphonylureas.[3]

Dosage

See Table 9.1.

Adverse effects

Hypoglycaemia

Sulphonylurea-induced hypoglycaemia, although rare, slower in onset and less severe than insulin-induced hypoglycaemia, is still a significant adverse effect and a medical emergency. The severity and frequency of hypoglycaemia is relatively more common with the longer-acting sulphonylureas such as chlorpropamide and glibenclamide. The risk of sulphonylurea-induced hypoglycaemia is greater in the elderly (use of short-acting sulphonylureas recommended) and in hepatic or renal impairment. Tolazamide, chlorpropamide and glibenclamide can cause significant hypoglycaemia in renal insufficiency due to the accumulation of the parent drug or active metabolites. The metabolites of tolbutamide, glipizide, gliclazide and gliquidone are either inactive or have minimal hypoglycaemic potency and therefore are less likely to cause hypoglycaemia in renal insufficiency. The use of the shorter-acting sulphonylureas with a reduction in dosage is recommended in renal impairment. The use of sulphonylureas in severe hepatic impairment is not recommended.[4] Drugs such as aspirin, sulphonamides and trimethoprim, which compete with sulphonylureas for binding to plasma albumin, have also been implicated in severe sulphonylurea-induced hypoglycaemia. There is an important difference between sulphonylurea-induced hypoglycaemia and insulin-induced hypoglycaemia. In sulphonylurea-induced hypoglycaemia, there are high levels of both insulin and sulphonylurea. Stimulation of insulin secretion by sulphonylurea continues until the drug is either metabolised or excreted. Treatment with intravenous glucose should be maintained until the sulphonylurea is cleared. Diazoxide or octreotide have been used to inhibit insulin secretion in cases of persistent sulphonylurea-induced hyperinsulinaemia. Treatment with glucagon is inappropriate as it can induce endogenous insulin release.

Cardiovascular effects

An increase in risk of cardiovascular disease has been reported with tolbutamide in the University Group Diabetes Program (UGDP) study.[5] The study design and interpretation of results have subsequently been criticised, and other studies have not provided supportive evidence. There is no significant effect on serum lipids. A small reduction in serum triglycerides has been reported with improved glycaemic control.[6] No evidence of adverse cardiovascular effects has been found with intensive treatment with chlorpropamide or glibenclamide.[7]

Weight gain

Sulphonylurea therapy can induce weight gain by reducing blood glucose concentrations (and hence glucosuria) in all patients who do not have absolute insulin deficiency. In patients who are unable to observe restrictions in their dietary intake, weight gain is inevitable as calorie loss (from glucosuria) is reduced without the corresponding reduction in calorie intake combined with the anabolic effects of increased insulin levels. The short- and medium-acting sulphonylureas may promote weight gain if the patients become hypoglycaemic around lunch-time.

Chlorpropamide-induced hyponatraemia (rare)

This is water retention due to sensitisation, by chlorpropamide, of the renal collecting ducts to the action of vasopressin. This may be exacerbated by concurrent use of thiazide diuretics, particularly in the elderly. In contrast, glibenclamide and tolazamide have a mild diuretic action.[8]

Other side effects

Other side effects include gastrointestinal disturbances, headache, and facial flushing after drinking alcohol (chlorpropamide).

Drug interactions

Hypoglycaemic effect enhanced

The hypoglycaemic effect of sulphonylureas can be enhanced by drugs that stimulate insulin secretion and those that enhance insulin action and glucose utilisation. The hypoglycaemic effect can also be enhanced by inhibition of sulphonylurea metabolism (by liver disease or drugs that inhibit liver enzymes) and excretion (by renal impairment or drugs that affect the renal clearance of a sulphonylurea or its metabolite).[9–11]

ACE inhibitors

See p. 94.

Alcohol

Flushing, headache, dizziness, nausea and vomiting may occur in those taking chlorpropamide. For a discussion on alcohol and hypoglycaemia, see p. 42.

Allopurinol

Marked hypoglycaemia in one patient on gliclazide has been reported, but the mechanism is not understood. An effect on the elimination half-life of chlorpropamide (increased) and tolbutamide (decreased) has also been reported but its clinical significance is uncertain. It may be prudent to monitor blood glucose levels when allopurinol therapy is initiated.

Antacids

The rate of absorption of sulphonylureas is increased by antacids containing magnesium hydroxide or sodium bicarbonate. A small increase in gastric pH may increase the solubility of sulphonylurea tablets and therefore their absorption. The effect on glibenclamide is dependent on whether the tablet formulation is micronised (not affected) or non-micronised (affected by antacids containing magnesium hydroxide and sodium bicarbonate). Transient hypoglycaemia may occur with glipizide/sodium bicarbonate, glipizide/magnesium hydroxide and tol-butamide/magnesium hydroxide (effect of tolbutamide increased 4-fold). These effects may be minimised by separating the doses of the antacid and sulphonylurea.

Anticoagulants

There is an established interaction between dicoumarol and tol-butamide, which mutually interact to enhance both the hypoglycaemic effect of tolbutamide (inhibition of metabolism by the liver) and the anti-coagulant effect of dicoumarol (displacement of plasma protein binding). Isolated reports of an enhanced hypoglycaemic effect of chlor-propamide with nicoumalone and an increased anticoagulant effect of warfarin with glibenclamide and tolbutamide.

Azapropazone

The effect of tolbutamide is increased, possibly by displacement from plasma proteins and inhibition of liver enzymes. Information on other sulphonylureas is lacking. It may be advisable to avoid concomitant use of azapropazone and tolbutamide.

Beta-blockers

Patients should be warned of the absence of some of the early 'adren-ergic' signs of hypoglycaemia. For effects on hypoglycaemic awareness, see pp. 94–96; for effects on insulin release, see Management Focus, p. 29.

Chloramphenicol

Hypoglycaemic effects of tolbutamide and chlorpropamide are increased, possibly by inhibition of liver enzyme activities. Information on other sulphonylureas is not available. A reduction in sulphonylurea dosage is probably required if chloramphenicol is used concomitantly.

Cimetidine

Isolated reports of hypoglycaemia when used with gliclazide and glipizide, possibly through the inhibition of sulphonylurea metabolism by the liver. It may be prudent to warn the patient of the possibility of hypoglycaemia occurring when cimetidine therapy is first started.

Co-trimoxazole (sulphamethoxazole and trimethoprim)

Hypoglycaemia has been reported in diabetic patients on glibenclamide, but the mechanism of interaction is not understood. No consistent pharmacokinetic interaction between glibenclamide and co-trimoxazole has been found, and hypoglycaemia has been reported with co-trimoxazole in diabetic patients who are not taking a sulphonylurea. The hypoglycaemic effect of co-trimoxazole may be due to the direct hypoglycaemic action of either sulphamethoxazole or trimethoprim.

Erythromycin

Isolated cases of hypoglycaemia with glibenclamide and severe hepatic damage with chlorpropamide have been reported. The mechanism is not understood. Patients should be closely monitored if erythromycin is used concomitantly with a sulphonylurea.

Fibrates

Effects of sulphonylureas are enhanced with clofibrate, possibly due to the direct lipid-lowering effect of clofibrate on glucose tolerance combined with the inhibition of sulphonylurea metabolism. Bezafibrate, ciprofibrate, fenofibrate and gemfibrozil also improve glucose tolerance, and severe hypoglycaemia in a few patients taking sulphonylureas has been reported. Monitor blood glucose levels closely; the dose of sulphonylurea may need to be reduced.

Fluconazole and miconazole

Plasma concentrations of sulphonylureas are increased, possibly by the inhibition of metabolism by the liver. Monitor patients closely, and warn them of the possibility of hypoglycaemia; the dose of sulphonylurea may need to be reduced.

Phenylbutazone

Sulphonylurea metabolism is inhibited. Monitor patients closely; the dose of sulphonylurea may need to be reduced.

Salicylates

In addition to direct glucose-lowering effects (see pp. 96–97), salicylates may interfere with the renal excretion of sulphonylureas. Aspirin can increase serum chlorpropamide levels, and severe hypoglycaemia following topical salicylic acid treatment, in a patient stabilised on glibenclamide, has been reported.[12]

Other interactions

Cholestyramine

Absorption of glipizide reduced.

Drugs impairing glucose tolerance

See Management Focus, p. 29.

Preparations

See Table 9.1.

References

1. Bailey C J. Hypoglycaemic, antihyperglycaemic and antidiabetic drugs. *Diabetes Care* 1992; 12: 553–564.
2. Scheen A J. Drug treatment of non-insulin-dependent diabetes mellitus in the 1990s. Achievements and future developments. *Drugs* 1997; 54: 355–368.
3. Hoechst Marion Roussel UK. *Amaryl. Summary of Product Characteristics.* November 1996.
4. Harrower A D B. Pharmacokinetics of oral antihyperglycaemic agents in patients with renal insufficiency. *Clin Pharmacokinet* 1996; 31: 111–119.
5. University Group Diabetes Program (UGDP). A study of the effects of hypoglycaemic agents on vascular complications in patients with adult-onset diabetes. *Diabetes* 1976; 25: 1129–1153.
6. Groop L C. Sulfonylureas in NIDDM. *Diabetes Care* 1992; 15: 737–754.
7. UK Prospective Diabetes Study (UKPDS) Group. Intensive blood-glucose control with sulphonylureas or insulin compared with conventional treatment

and risk of complications in patients with type 2 diabetes (UKPDS 33). *Lancet* 1998, 352: 837–853.

8. Krentz A J, Ferner R E, Bailey C J. Comparative tolerability profiles of oral antidiabetic agents. *Drug Safety* 1994; 11: 223–241.

9. Stockley I H. *Drug Interactions*, 4th edition. London: Pharmaceutical Press, 1996.

10. Scheen A J, Lefebvre P J. Antihyperglycaemic agents. Drug interactions of clinical importance. *Drug Safety* 1995; 12: 32–45.

11. Ferner R E. Drug-induced hypoglycaemia. *Adverse Drug Reaction Bulletin* 1996; No. 179: 679–682.

12. Maurer T A, Winter M E, Koo J, *et al*. Refractory hypoglycaemia: a complication of topical salicylate therapy. *Arch Dermatol* 1994; 130: 1455–1457.

10

Metformin

Indications

Metformin is used for the management of type 2 diabetes mellitus when dietary management alone has failed. Metformin is particularly useful for the management of obese type 2 diabetic patients; it may be used as monotherapy or in combination with a sulphonylurea (see Chapter 7).

Mechanism of action

The biguanides were developed from a traditional plant remedy, *Galege officinalis* (French lilac, goat's rue). Guanidine was identified in 1918 as the plant component exhibiting mild antidiabetic activity. Guanidine itself was too toxic for clinical use, and the two biguanide derivatives – phenformin and metformin – were developed in the 1950s (see Figure 10.1). Phenformin undergoes metabolism via hydroxylation before being excreted. A small percentage of the Caucasian population has a hereditary defect that affects the hydroxylation process and which increases the risk of accumulation of the drug due to inadequate

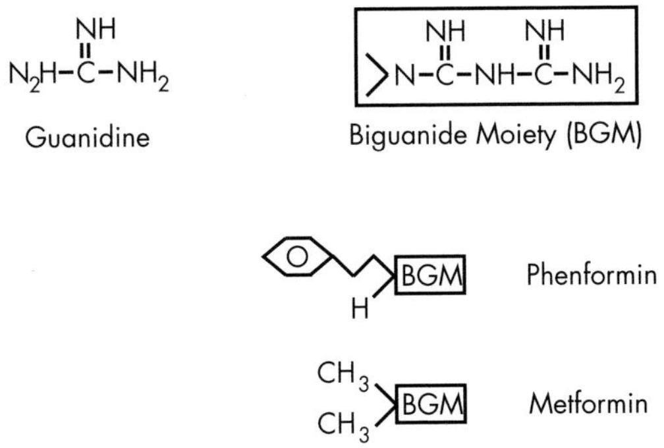

Figure 10.1 Biguanides.

metabolism. Phenformin also inhibits peripheral glucose oxidation and enhances peripheral lactate production. The association of phenformin with the potentially lethal side effect, lactic acidosis, led to its withdrawal from clinical use in the UK. It is still available for the treatment of type 2 diabetes in some countries such at Italy and Spain. Metformin is the only biguanide in clinical use in the UK.[1]

Metformin increases insulin sensitivity and is only effective in the presence of insulin. It reduces blood glucose levels mainly by increasing glucose utilisation. Metformin enhances insulin action at the post-receptor level in peripheral tissues such as muscle where it increases insulin-mediated glucose uptake (possibly by increasing the number of glucose transporters, GLUT4; see pp. 82–83) and oxidative metabolism. Metformin acts as an 'antihyperglycaemic' agent rather than a 'hypoglycaemic' agent. It increases the intestinal use of glucose via non-oxidative metabolism which results in the production of lactate. The lactate is extracted by the liver where it serves as a substrate for gluconeogenesis and provides a safeguard against hypoglycaemia. There is also a decrease in hepatic glucose output which correlates with a decrease in fasting plasma glucose and an increase in peripheral glucose uptake. Metformin does not appear to enhance peripheral glucose uptake in the short term, but in the long term, improvement in glycaemic control leads to an increase in insulin sensitivity and an improvement in glucose uptake by peripheral tissues.[2–4]

Contraindications

The development of lactic acidosis with metformin has been associated with the presence of concomitant conditions (see Adverse Effects Focus opposite). These conditions are regarded as cautions or contraindications to metformin therapy. Regular monitoring for renal impairment, which would increase the plasma concentration of metformin (see under Pharmacokinetics and Drug Interactions, below) or for any condition that would disturb lactate metabolism, is advisable for patients on metformin therapy.[5,6] Substitution with insulin therapy is recommended in medical or surgical emergencies and also before elective surgery.[7]

Pharmacokinetics

Gastrointestinal absorption of metformin is complete within 6 h of ingestion (oral bioavailability 40–60%). Metformin does not bind to plasma proteins, and no metabolites or conjugates have been identified.

ADVERSE EFFECTS FOCUS

Contraindications for metformin therapy

- Renal impairment (an absolute contraindication if serum creatinine >130 μmol/L or in those at risk of sudden deterioration of renal function)
- Hepatic impairment (including alcoholic liver disease)
- Predisposition to lactic acidosis or history of lactic acidosis
- Cardiac or respiratory insufficiency (likely to cause hypoxia or reduced peripheral perfusion)
- Severe infection or trauma (could lead to decreased tissue perfusion)
- Dehydration (could lead to reduced peripheral perfusion)
- Alcohol dependence (alcohol abuse with binge drinking sufficient to cause hepatic toxicity; moderate alcohol intake is not a contraindication, if liver function is normal)

Excretion is via the kidneys with a mean plasma elimination half-life after oral administration of 4–9 h. Elimination is prolonged in patients with renal impairment and correlates with creatinine clearance. Monitoring of plasma metformin has little clinical value unless lactic acidosis is suspected or present. If lactic acidosis is confirmed, the drug can be rapidly eliminated by forced diuresis or haemodialysis.[8,9]

Dosage

This is usually 500 mg every 8 h or 850 mg every 12 h with or after food. The maximum dose is 3 g daily in divided doses (a maximum of 2 g is preferable because of the greater incidence of gastrointestinal disturbances at high doses).

Adverse effects

Lactic acidosis

Metformin is excreted unchanged in the urine. It does not affect peripheral glucose oxidation and peripheral lactate production in the same way as phenformin. Metformin therapy causes a small increase in postprandial blood lactate which is probably due to metformin-induced conversion of glucose to lactate by the intestinal mucosa. The lactate then enters the portal circulation and is largely cleared by the liver in which it serves as a gluconeogenic substrate. Most of the reported occurrences of lactic acidosis with metformin have been due to factors which either lead to high plasma concentrations of metformin (e.g. occurring in renal impairment) or where there is an increase in blood lactate concentrations (such as in liver disease, alcohol abuse or an illness causing hypotension, which leads to a decrease in tissue perfusion and hypoxia). Lactic acidosis can be avoided if conditions such as renal impairment are excluded before initiating metformin therapy.[5] If a metformin-treated patient has a serious illness where there is a substantial rise in blood lactate, deterioration of renal function, impaired hepatic function, deterioration of cardiovascular function or any condition where metformin is contraindicated (see Adverse Effects Focus, p. 115), it is advisable to transfer the patient on to insulin at least until the patient has fully recovered.

Other side effects

Transient and dose-related side effects are seen in up to 20% of patients and include diarrhoea and other gastrointestinal disturbances such as abdominal discomfort, nausea and metallic taste. These effects can be minimised by increasing the dose slowly and taking the tablets after food. Absorption of vitamin B_{12} and folate is often decreased on long-term therapy, but this effect rarely causes clinical problems.

Drug interactions

Risk of lactic acidosis increased

Drugs that impair renal function may affect the renal excretion of metformin, and concomitant use can lead to the development of lactic acidosis. Co-administration of drugs that reduce renal excretion of metformin and, in particular, drugs that impair renal function should be avoided, particularly in the elderly. When this is not possible, a reduction in metformin dosage or discontinuation of metformin therapy should be considered.[10–12]

Alcohol

Isolated cases of potentiation of lactic acidosis has been reported. Moderate alcohol intake where liver function is normal does not appear to be a problem (see Adverse Effects Focus, p. 115). For a discussion on alcohol and hypoglycaemia, see p. 42.

Cimetidine

Increases bioavailability and reduces renal excretion of metformin. The dose of metformin may need to be reduced (particularly in the elderly).

Iodine preparations (used in radiology)

Excreted in the urine and temporarily impairs renal function.

Other interactions

Acarbose

Significantly reduces bioavailability of metformin. Clinical significance in type 2 diabetic patients treated with a combination of metformin and acarbose is not established.

Guar gum

Significantly reduces the rate of absorption and blood metformin levels up to 6 h after administration in healthy volunteers. Data for the diabetic population are not available.

Drugs impairing glucose tolerance

See Management Focus, p. 29.

Preparations

See Table 9.1.

References

1. Nattrass M (ed.). *Malin's Clinical Diabetes*, 2nd edition. London: Chapman & Hall, 1996.
2. Bailey C J. Biguanides and NIDDM. *Diabetes Care* 1992; 15: 755–772.
3. Klip A, Leiter L A. Cellular mechanism of action of metformin. *Diabetes Care* 1990; 13: 696–708.
4. Hermann L S, Melander A. Biguanides: basic aspects and clinical uses. In: Alberti K G M M, DeFronzo R A, Keen H, Zimmet P, eds. *International Textbook of Diabetes Mellitus*. Chichester: John Wiley & Sons, 1992: 773–795.
5. Salpeter S, Greyber E, Pasternek G, Salpeter E. Risk of fatal and non-fatal lactic acidosis with metformin use in type 2 diabetes mellitus. The Cochrane Library, Issue 3, 2002. Oxford: Update Software.

6. Royal College of General Practitioners Effective Clinical Practice Unit. Clinical Guidelines for Type 2 Diabetes: Management of Blood Glucose, 2002. www.nice.org.uk (last accessed December 2002).

7. Sulkin T U, Bosman D, Krenlz A J. Contraindications to metformin therapy in patients with NIDDM. *Diabetes Care* 1997; 20: 925–928.

8. Bailey C, Turner M D. Metformin. *N Engl J Med* 1996; 334: 574–579.

9. Scheen A J. Clinical pharmacokinetics of metformin. *Clin Pharmacokinet* 1996; 30: 359–371.

10. Stockley I H. *Drug Interactions*, 4th edition. London: Pharmaceutical Press, 1996.

11. Scheen A J, Lefebvre P J. Antihyperglycaemic agents. Drug interactions of clinical importance. *Drug Safety* 1995; 12: 32–45.

12. Ferner R E. Drug-induced hypoglycaemia. *Adverse Drug Reaction Bulletin* 1996; No. 179: 679–682.

11

Acarbose

Indications

Acarbose is used in combination with other antidiabetic drugs for reducing post-prandial hyperglycaemia (see Chapter 7).

Mechanism of action

Acarbose is a reversible competitive inhibitor of alpha-glucosidase enzymes (particularly sucrase) which are located in the brush border of the small intestine and are responsible for breaking down non-absorbable complex carbohydrates into absorbable monosaccharides. It is a pseudo-tetrasaccharide which structurally resembles typical oligosaccharides derived from starch digestion (see Figure 11.1). The acarbose molecule consists of two components: acarviosine (substituted cyclohexene ring and 4,6-dideoxy-4-amino-D-glucose unit), which binds to the active site of the enzyme preventing cleavage of the substrate, and

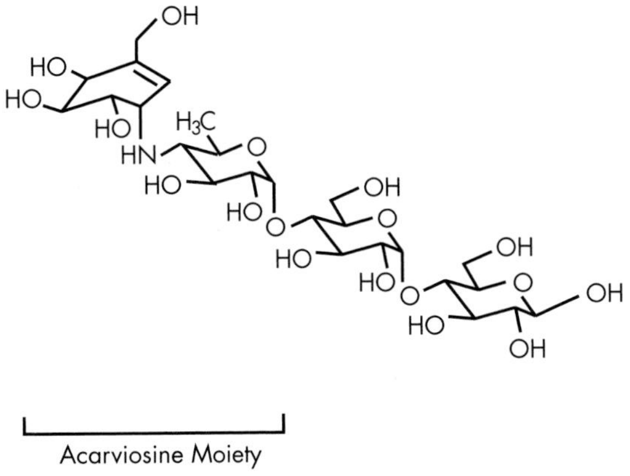

Acarbose

Acarviosine Moiety

Figure 11.1   Acarbose.

a two-glucose unit, which determines the specificity of acarbose for the enzyme.[1]

Acarbose blunts and delays the peak rise in post-prandial blood glucose by inhibiting carbohydrate digestion and slowing down the absorption of monosaccharides. The carbohydrates that are not digested in the upper part of the small intestine are transported to the ileum where the digestive process may be completed. If the dose of acarbose is sufficient to overcome carbohydrate digestive capacity, undigested carbohydrate will enter the colon where it is hydrolysed through bacterial activity, which causes dose-dependent gastrointestinal discomfort. The effect of acarbose on post-prandial plasma glucose levels depends on the carbohydrate composition of meals. Acarbose has no effect on monosaccharides, e.g. glucose, fructose and sorbitol, which are directly absorbed, or carbohydrates which are not digestible e.g. lactulose, or which are not cleaved by alpha-glucosidases e.g. lactose (see Table 6.1, pp. 60–61).[1,2]

Pharmacokinetics

Acarbose does not cross the intestinal microvillar membrane. It is transported through the intestinal tract into the colon where degradation occurs via two pathways: (i) the acarbose molecule is split into two components; and (ii) a complex mixture of acidic metabolites are formed via a sequence of biotransformation reactions which are dependent on the microbial content of the colon. Around 35% of the metabolites (which are inactive) are slowly absorbed and then rapidly eliminated by renal excretion.[1,2]

Dosage

In order to reduce gastrointestinal side effects, a low starting dose of 50 mg daily is recommended. This may gradually be increased to 50 mg three times daily and then increased further, if necessary, after 6–8 weeks to 100 mg three times daily. The maximum dose is 200 mg three times daily (see Adverse Effects, below).

Adverse effects

Gastrointestinal disturbances such as flatulence, abdominal distension and diarrhoea are dose-dependent and caused by the presence of undigested carbohydrate in the large intestine. Adverse effects tend to decrease with time and appear to be due to an adaptive process of carbo-hydrate digestion. Therefore the incidence of these effects can be reduced by starting with a low dose and gradually increasing it at 4-weekly intervals.[1,3]

Hypoglycaemia

Acarbose itself does not cause hypoglycaemia, but may enhance the effects of either insulin (see pp. 92–93) or sulphonylureas (see pp. 106–107). The absorption of sucrose is affected by acarbose (see pp. 119–120); therefore it is necessary to use glucose rather than sucrose to counteract any symptoms of hypoglycaemia (see Adverse Effects Focus, p. 37; see also Table 6.1, pp. 60–61).

Drug interactions

Drugs affecting the action of acarbose[4,5]

Cholestyramine

May enhance the effects of acarbose on post-prandial blood glucose.

Neomycin

May enhance effect of acarbose on post-prandial blood glucose and increase the severity of gastrointestinal disturbances.

Pancreatin and charcoal

May decrease the effect of acarbose.

Drugs impairing glucose tolerance

See Management Focus, p. 29.

Preparations

See Table 9.1.

References

1.   Salvatore T, Giugliano D. Pharmacokinetic–pharmacodynamic relationships of acarbose. *Clin Pharmacokinet* 1996; 30: 94–104.

2.   Bailey C J. Hypoglycaemic, antihyperglycaemic and antidiabetic drugs. *Diabetes Care* 1992; 12: 553–564.

3.   Johnson A B, Taylor R. Drugs in focus: 19. Acarbose. *Prescribers' Journal* 1996; 36: 169–172.

4.   Stockley I H. *Drug Interactions*, 4th edition. London: Pharmaceutical Press, 1996.

5.   Scheen A J, Lefebvre P J. Antihyperglycaemic agents. Drug interactions of clinical importance. *Drug Safety* 1995; 12: 32–45.

12

Thiazolidinediones (PPAR-γ-agonists)

Indications

Thiazolidinediones (Figure 12.1) are a new class of drugs known as the peroxisome proliferator-activated receptor-gamma (PPAR-γ) agonists. Two thiazolidinediones, pioglitazone and rosiglitazone, are currently licensed in the UK for use in combination with metformin or a sulphonylurea for the management of type 2 diabetes when combination therapy with metformin plus a sulphonylurea has failed (see Chapter 7).

Mechanism of action

Thiazolidinediones lower blood glucose levels by increasing insulin sensitivity mainly in skeletal muscle and adipose tissue. Therefore, the action of reducing blood glucose levels is dependent on the presence of endogenous insulin. Thiazolidinediones increase insulin sensitivity in skeletal muscle and adipose tissue by increasing glucose utilisation (increased glucose uptake and glycolysis and normalisation of insulin receptor functions). It reduces hepatic glucose output (HGO) by increasing glucose uptake and glycogen synthesis and reducing gluconeogenesis. There is also an overall decrease in circulating insulin and plasma triglyceride levels in type 2 diabetic patients. Thiazolidinediones require the presence of insulin in order to reduce blood glucose levels and so do not directly cause hypoglycaemia. The precise mechanism of molecular action of thiazolidinediones has yet to be established, but may involve interaction with nuclear receptors that regulate gene expression. Insulin-sensitising effects of thiazolidinediones do not appear to involve any early signalling events of insulin action. Studies conducted so far indicate that the primary insulin-sensitising effect may be mediated through regulation of transcription in fat cells.

Thiazolidinediones induce adipocyte differentiation by interacting with peroxisome PPARs, which are members of the steroid and thyroid hormone receptor superfamily of transcription factors. Three subtypes of PPAR – α, γ and δ – have been identified. Although it has been

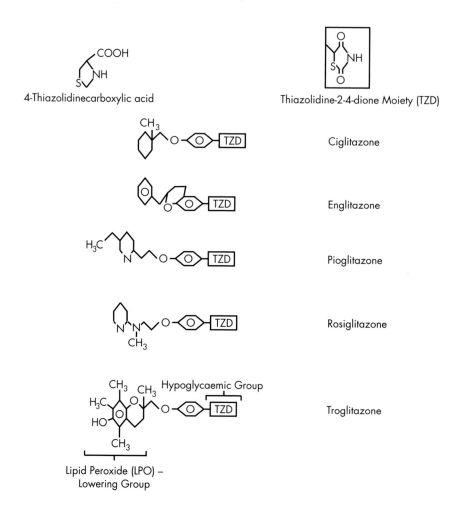

4-Thiazolidinecarboxylic acid

Thiazolidine-2-4-dione Moiety (TZD)

Ciglitazone

Englitazone

Pioglitazone

Rosiglitazone

Troglitazone

Lipid Peroxide (LPO) –
Lowering Group

Figure 12.1   Thiazolidinediones (PPAR-γ-agonists).

suggested that the interaction of thiazolidinediones is mainly with PPAR-γ, the relative roles of the three subtypes remains uncertain.[1–3]

Ciglitazone was the first thiazolidinedione derivative to be discovered in the early 1980s. This has been followed by the development of other derivatives including troglitazone, pioglitazone, rosiglitazone and englitazone.[1] Troglitazone, the first in this class of compounds to be licensed for the management of type 2 diabetes, was designed to exhibit both antihyperglycaemic and lipid peroxide (LPO) lowering properties (see Figure 12.1). The lipid peroxide-lowering property of the compound is provided by an α-tocopherol (antioxidant) substituent in the molecule. Lipid peroxides contribute to the development of atherosclerosis by oxidising unsaturated fatty acids in low-density lipoproteins (LDL), mainly in the arterial wall.[2] Troglitazone and pioglitazone have partial PPAR-α agonist activity, which may explain why troglitazone and pioglitazone lower serum triglycerides whereas rosiglitazone, which does not have PPAR-α agonist activity, does not lower serum triglycerides.[3–5]

Contraindications

Heart failure

Thiazolidinediones have been associated with increased plasma volume and peripheral oedema. Thiazolidinediones are contraindicated in people with a history of heart failure. The combination with exogenous insulin is also not recommended because of the risk of heart failure.[6,7]

Pharmacokinetics

Both rosiglitazone and pioglitazone are rapidly absorbed and extensively bound to plasma proteins. Rosiglitazone is completely metabolised in the liver via the cytochrome P450 isoform CYP2C8 enzyme, producing metabolites with weak activity, and is eliminated via the urine. Pioglitazone is metabolised by several P450 isoforms including CYP2C8 and CYP3A4, producing active metabolites, and is eliminated mainly in the bile.[8]

Dosage

See Table 9.1.

Adverse effects

Initial deterioration in glycaemic control

Control of blood glucose may deteriorate initially when metformin or a sulphonylurea is replaced with a thiazolidindione in combination therapy because of the slow onset of effect of thiazolidinediones.

Cardiovascular effects

Rosiglitazone is associated with a significant increase in serum LDL-cholesterol and total cholesterol, while HDL-cholesterol levels are only slightly increased. However, pioglitazone seems to significantly increase HDL-cholesterol levels within the first 24 weeks of treatment while not significantly affecting LDL-cholesterol and total cholesterol levels.[6]

Liver failure

Troglitazone was licensed for use in type 2 diabetes in 1997 (USA and Japan, March 1997; UK, October 1997).[9] Owing to world-wide reports of serious hepatic reactions (hepatocellular damage, hepatic necrosis and hepatic failure), troglitazone (*Romozin*) has since been withdrawn.[10] The risk factors for the development of these hepatic reactions have not been established. Pioglitazone and rosiglitazone do not appear to have the problem of hepatic toxicity, but liver enzyme monitoring is recommended before initiation of treatment, every two months for the first year, and at regular intervals thereafter.[6,7]

Weight gain

An increase in body weight of around 3–4 kg has been reported in the first year of treatment with thiazolidinediones. Weight gain is less when thiazolidinediones are used in combination with metformin. The increase in weight seems to be largely due to an increase in subcutaneous fat deposits rather than an increase in visceral fat and up to 0.5 kg may be due to fluid retention.[6,8]

Other side effects

Other side effects include gastrointestinal disturbances, headache, visual disturbances, proteinuria, decreased haematocrit and haemoglobin.

Drug interactions

No clinically relevant interactions with other drugs have yet been reported.

Drugs impairing glucose tolerance

See Management Focus, p. 29.

Preparations

See Table 9.1.

References

1. Saltiel A R, Olefsky J M. Thiazolidinediones in the treatment of insulin resistance and type II diabetes. *Diabetes* 1996; 45: 1661–1669.
2. Horikoshi H, Yoshioka T. Troglitazone – a novel antidiabetic drug for treating insulin resistance. *Drug Discovery Today* 1998; 3: 79–88.
3. Chehade J M, Arshag D M. A rational approach to drug therapy of type 2 diabetes mellitus. *Drugs* 2000; 60: 95–113.
4. Gillies P S, Dunn C J. Pioglitazone. *Drugs* 2000; 60: 333–343.
5. Barman Balfour J A, Plosker G L. Rosiglitazone. *Drugs* 1999; 57: 921–930.
6. Campbell I W. Antidiabetic drugs present and future. Will improving insulin resistance benefit cardiovascular risk in type 2 diabetes mellitus? *Drugs* 2000; 60: 1017–1028.
7. The Royal College of General Practitioners Effective Clinical Practice Unit. Clinical Guidelines for Management of Type 2 Diabetes: Management of Blood Glucose. 2002. www.nice.org.uk (last accessed December 2002).
8. Bailey C J, Day C. Thiazolidinediones today. *Br J Diabetes Vasc Dis* 2001; 1: 7–13.
9. GlaxoWellcome. *Romozin Tablets*. Summary of product characteristics. July 1997.
10. CSM Current Problems in Pharmacovigilance. Troglitazone (Romozin) withdrawn. *Curr Probl* 1997; December: 23.

13

Meglitinides

Indications

Meglitinides (Figure 13.1) are a new chemical class of insulin secret-agogue drugs. Two meglitinide analogues, nateglinide and repaglinide, are currently licensed in the UK for use in the management of type 2 diabetes. Nateglinide is licensed for use only in combination with metformin, whereas repaglinide may be used either as monotherapy or in combination with metformin (see Chapter 7).

Mechanism of action

Meglitinides stimulates insulin release by pancreatic beta-cells by closing ATP-dependent potassium channels in a similar way to sulphonylureas, but binds with different receptor sites compared with the sulphonyl-ureas.[1,2] Repaglinide was the first meglitinide to be developed from the

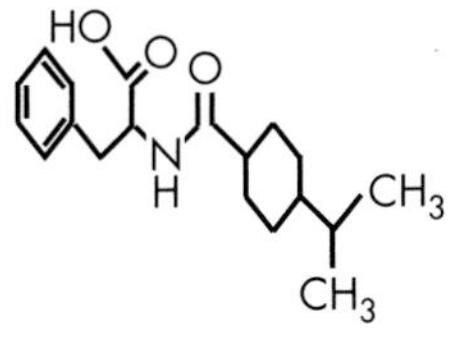

Nateglinide

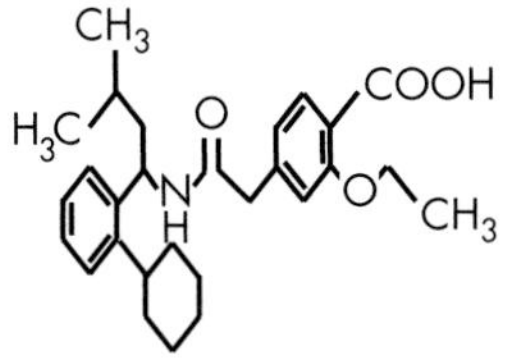

Repaglinide

Figure 13.1   Meglitinides.

non-sulphonylurea part of the glibenclamide molecule (see Figure 9.1, p. 104).[3,4] Unlike the sulphonylureas, repaglinide does not appear to cause direct exocytosis of glucagon.

Pharmacokinetics

Both nateglinide and repaglinide have a rapid onset and short duration of action, and therefore can be administered shortly before a meal. Nateglinide is rapidly absorbed after oral administration, with peak plasma concentrations occurring within an hour. It is mainly metabolised by the cytochrome P450 isoenzyme CYP2C9, and to a lesser extent by CYP3A4. Nateglinide and its metabolites are mainly excreted in the urine, and about 10% is eliminated in the faeces. Repaglinide is also rapidly absorbed after oral administration, with peak plasma concentrations occurring within an hour. It is metabolised in the liver by the cytochrome P450 isoenzyme CYP3A4 to inactive metabolites which are excreted in the bile.

Dosage

See Table 9.1.

Adverse effects

Hypoglycaemia

Both nateglinide and repaglinide can cause hypoglycaemia in a similar way to the shorter-acting sulphonylureas

Weight gain

Both nateglinide and repaglinide can cause weight gain in a similar way to the shorter-acting sulphonylureas

Other side effects

Other side effects of meglitinides include diarrhoea, constipation, nausea, vomiting and transient elevations in liver enzyme activities

Drug interactions

No clinically relevant interactions with other drugs have yet been reported.

Drugs impairing glucose tolerance

See Management Focus, p. 29.

Preparations

See Table 9.1.

References

1. Graul A, Castaner J. Repaglinide. *Drugs Future* 1996; 21: 694–699.
2. Dunn C J, Faulds D. Nateglinide. *Drugs* 2000; 60: 607–615.
3. Fuhlendroff J, Rorsman P, Kofod H, *et al*. Stimulation of insulin release by repaglinide and glibenclamide involves both common and distinct process. *Diabetes* 1998; 47: 345–351.
4. Campbell I W. Antidiabetic drugs present and future: will improving insulin resistance benefit cardiovascular risk in Type 2 diabetes mellitus? *Drugs* 2000; 60: 1017–1028.

14

New therapies and future developments

Amylin analogues

Under normal physiological conditions, amylin – a hormone – modulates the action of insulin by regulating the absorption of glucose from the gastrointestinal tract. It has been suggested that administration of amylin-like substances may improve glycaemic control in diabetic patients treated with insulin. Pramlintide, a synthetic analogue of amylin, has been shown to reduce glycosylated haemoglobin, though the degree of reduction is modest.[1] Pramlintide is being evaluated in clinical trials for control of post-prandial hyperglycaemia in both type 1 and type 2 diabetes.

Glucagon-like peptide-1

Glucagon-like peptide-1 (GLP-1) is an incretin that has insulin-like effect (possibly through inhibition of glucagon) and inhibits gastric emptying. It has been shown to reduce post-prandial hyperglycaemia in type 2 diabetic patients after either intravenous or subcutaneous administration. GLP-1, which is a fragment of the proglucagon molecule, does not cause hypoglycaemia as it requires the presence of glucose in order to stimulate insulin release from pancreatic beta-cells. The drawbacks of GLP-1 as an antidiabetic agent for type 2 diabetes are its short duration of action and the requirement for parenteral administration.[2]

Miglitol

The structure of miglitol is similar to that of glucose. Like acarbose, it inhibits gastrointestinal alpha-glucosidase enzymes (see pp. 119–120) but, unlike acarbose, it is completely absorbed. Miglitol has been shown to reduce post-prandial hyperglycaemia in type 2 diabetic patients, this effect being independent of the starch content of the meal. Miglitol may be useful as an adjunct to diet or sulphonylurea therapy in type 2 diabetes.[2] Voglibose is another alpha-glucosidase inhibitor.

New formulations for insulin

Insulin is administered mainly by subcutaneous injection, and although this route is 'successful' in terms of insulin delivery, it is generally not ideal because of the inconvenience caused to the individual with diabetes and the variability in insulin absorption. The search for new formulations of insulin with non-parenteral administration has been underway for some time, but this is a challenging problem because insulin as a polypeptide cannot cross the mucosal membranes without the assistance of absorption-promoting agents. The non-invasive routes for insulin administration which have been investigated include nasal, ocular, buccal, rectal, pulmonary, oral and transdermal.

To date, with the exception of the pulmonary route, all the alternative routes of insulin administration have failed due to poor and variable insulin bioavailability.[3]

The pulmonary route for insulin delivery seems promising following the development of inhalation devices capable of consistently generating insulin small-sized particles. The bioavailability of inhaled insulin is low (10–20%) however, with 80–90% of the administered dose being lost through exhalation. The benefits of inhaled insulin over subcutaneous administration of insulin remain to be proven.[4]

References

1. Gibaldi M. New approaches to drug therapy. *Pharm News* 1998; 5: 32–33.
2. Scheen A J. Drug treatment of non-insulin dependent diabetes mellitus in the 1990s. Achievements and future developments. *Drugs* 1997; 54: 355–368.
3. Hoffman A, Ziv E. Pharmacokinetic considerations of new insulin formulations and routes of administration. *Clin Pharmacokinet* 1997; 33: 285–301.
4. Barnett A H. Completing the revolution – towards sustained euglycaemia in insulin therapy. *Mod Diabetes Management* 2002; 3: 2–8.

15

Prevention of and screening for diabetes mellitus

Preventative strategies, implemented at three levels, have been used in an attempt to reduce the incidence of morbidity and mortality from diabetic complications.[1-4] The three levels of strategies include:

- *Primary prevention*: population-based strategy aimed at reducing the prevalence of diabetes mellitus.
- *Secondary prevention*: strategy to reduce the prevalence of complications following diagnosis of diabetes mellitus (see Chapter 3).
- *Tertiary prevention*: strategy to reduce progression of diabetic complications once they have developed (see Chapter 3).

This section deals with primary prevention of the disease and population screening for early diagnosis of diabetes mellitus.

Primary prevention of diabetes mellitus

At present, there is no clinical basis for interventions to prevent type 1 diabetes mellitus. Type 2 diabetes is the most prevalent form of diabetes mellitus and affects more than one million people in the UK.[5,6] Possibilities exist for the primary prevention of type 2 diabetes where potentially modifiable risk factors, associated with lifestyle, have been identified. Risk factors for type 2 diabetes mellitus are similar to those for cardiovascular disease (see Chapter 3). The potentially modifiable risk factors that influence insulin secretion and action include:

- Obesity (associated with insulin resistance and earlier onset of diabetes).
- Physical activity (associated with glucose uptake and effects on blood lipids profile).
- Dietary modification (the prevalence of diabetes has been associated with high fat intake).
- Smoking.

- Hypertension.
- Dyslipidaemia.

Whether a reduction in the number of modifiable risk factors prevents or delays the onset of type 2 diabetes remains to be established.

Population screening

The primary purpose of population-based screening is to detect the disease at an early stage with a view to improving the outcome through prevention of diabetic complications.[1] The rapid nature of the onset of type 1 diabetes means that few people remain undiagnosed for any length of time. Some people with type 1 diabetes can become ill very quickly and can develop diabetic ketoacidosis before they are diagnosed as having the condition. A high proportion of people with type 2 diabetes remain undiagnosed for several years. The management targets for prevention of diabetic complications include glycaemic control and a reduction in the number of risk factors for cardiovascular disease (see Chapter 3). There is now firm evidence that the progression of microvascular complications may be slowed down by good glycaemic control (see p. 12). It therefore seems reasonable to identify previously undiagnosed asymptomatic individuals with type 2 diabetes with the aim of reducing microvascular complications. The effects of early detection and treatment of diabetes on macrovascular complications are unknown.[7] However, targeting high-risk groups for screening for type 2 diabetes is a possible method for reducing the cost and complications of the condition. Population screening must take into account risk factors, signs and symptoms and the results of any screening test.

Risk factors for type 2 diabetes

The UK National Screening Committee has reviewed the evidence for population screening programmes that suggests that targeting high-risk groups may be appropriate.[8] High-risk groups have been defined as:

- Those with multiple risk factors for diabetes such as family history of diabetes in parent or sibling.
- Belonging to an ethnic group with a higher prevalence of diabetes (e.g. people from South Asian, African and African-Caribbean communities).

- Being overweight and obese or having a high waist circumference or waist–hip ratio (see Risk Factors Focus, p. 139).
- Being aged over 40 years.[8,9]

Signs and symptoms

If a person presents with any signs or symptoms of diabetes (see Risk Factors Focus, below), they should be advised to see a general practitioner for diagnostic testing in line with WHO recommendations (see Chapter 2).[8,10]

Screening methods

The test used for screening should ideally be sensitive and specific, as false-positive results can cause people unnecessary worry and false-negative results can give people a false sense of security and may delay the diagnosis of diabetes.[7] A screening test is not a diagnostic test, and

RISK FACTORS FOCUS

Signs and symptoms of diabetes mellitus

Symptoms:

- Increased thirst
- Passing a lot of urine, especially at night
- Extreme tiredness and lethargy
- Weight loss despite increased appetite
- Genital itching
- Itchy skin rash
- Discomfort or pain on passing urine
- Blurred vision
- Tingling, pain and numbness in feet, legs or hands
- Sore or burning mouth

Signs:

- Persistent or recurrent infections, such as skin infections, oral or genital thrush, mouth ulcers and urinary tract infections
- Cataracts
- Signs of microvascular complications such as retinopathy detected by an optometrist during routine eye check, foot ulcers, loss of sensation in lower limbs, or impotence (erectile dysfunction)
- Signs of cardiovascular disease such as high blood pressure, abnormal blood lipids, fatty deposits in the eyelids, absent foot pulses

Criteria for blood glucose screening in asymptomatic high-risk individuals*		
Blood glucose concentration (mmol/L)		
Normal	*Uncertain**	*Possible diabetes**
Random <5.6	5.6–11.0	≥11.1
Fasting <5.6	5.6–6.0	>6.1

Random (casual): defined as any time of the day without consideration being given to the lapse of time since the last meal.
Fasting: defined as no calorie intake for at least 8 h before the test.
*Referral to a General Practitioner recommended. Diagnosis must be confirmed by laboratory estimation of blood glucose according to the guidelines for diagnosis (see pp. 5–6).

*Adapted from Diabetes UK Care Recommendation. Early identification of diabetes for community pharmacists, August 2001. www.diabetes.org.uk (last accessed December 2002) and WHO Definition, Diagnosis and Classification of Diabetes Mellitus and its complications (Part 1). 1999.[11]

clinical diagnosis should not be based on glycosuria or blood glucose values detected by a 'dip-stick' or a 'finger-prick' test alone (see pp. 5–6). Results from such tests should only be used as indicators for further investigations (see Chapter 2).[10,11]

Random urine glucose

The sensitivity of this method for detection of diabetes is low. In elderly patients who have a tendency towards a high renal threshold for glucose, glucosuria may be undetected unless the blood glucose value exceeds 15 mmol/L (see pp. 48–50). A positive test indicates that further investigation is needed.

Random blood glucose

The main difficulty with using random blood glucose testing as a method for screening is in establishing a 'cut-off' figure for the test. Results are dependent on timing, food eaten before the test, and other factors such as stress and physical activity. If the 'cut-off' figure is set too low, there will be too many false positives, while if it is set too high there will be too many false negatives. The most effective time to carry out the test is

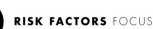

RISK FACTORS FOCUS

Diabetes UK questionnaire for identification of individuals at risk of type 2 diabetes*

- Are you aged over 40?
- Are you overweight?
- Do you have a family history of diabetes?
- Did you have diabetes during pregnancy?
- Have you had a baby that weighed over 4.5 kg (10 lb)?
- Are you Asian or African-Caribbean?

If you have answered yes to more than one question you may be at increased risk of diabetes. You need to know more about the symptoms of diabetes.

Symptoms of diabetes include:

- Feeling thirsty all the time
- Going to the loo a lot
- Feeling tired

If you are concerned, see your GP for advice.

---

*Adapted from the Diabetes UK leaflet *'Are you at risk of Diabetes?'*[12]

after a meal (1.5–2.0 h) or fasting (overnight from 10 p.m.; drinking water or tea without sugar is allowed) (see Screening Focus, above).[10,11]

Screening questionnaires

This method has the advantage of being non-invasive. It involves the distribution of a general questionnaire (see Risk Factors Focus, above) inviting members of the public to carry out a self-assessment for the risk of diabetes.[12,13] The aim of the questionnaire is to identify individuals with two or more risk factors and to alert them to the possibility of having diabetes in order that they seek medical help.

The diagnosis of diabetes carries significant lifelong consequences for the individual concerned. It is essential that appropriate interpretation of the test results is provided for the patient and that follow-up evaluation and treatment are available. Consideration must be given to other causes of hyperglycaemia, for example drugs such as glucocorticoids and thiazide diuretics which can affect glucose tolerance (see Management Focus, p. 29).

References

1. World Health Organization. *Prevention of Diabetes Mellitus: Report of a WHO Study Group*. Geneva: World Health Organization (Technical Report Series No. 844), 1994: 18–68.
2. Dornhorst A. Taking up the challenge: a practical approach to reducing the burden of type II diabetes. *Reducing the Burden of Diabetes*, Medical Action Communications Ltd, UK, 1995; Issue 1.
3. NHS Executive Health Service Guidelines. *Key Features of Good Diabetes Service*. Department of Health 1997; HSG (97): 45.
4. Waine C. *Diabetes in General Practice*, 3rd edition. RCGP Clinical Series. Royal College of General Practitioners, 1992.
5. O'Rahilly S. Science, medicine, and the future. Non-insulin dependent diabetes mellitus: the gathering storm. *Br Med J* 1997; 314: 955–959.
6. Bonney R. Dealing with the diabetes epidemic. *Scrip* 1995; December: 40–45.
7. Anonymous. Should population screening be conducted for non-insulin dependent diabetes? *Diabetes Update* 1996; Winter: 4–5.
8. Department of Health. National Service Framework for Diabetes: Standards 2002. Interventions.
9. Anonymous. Call to widen diabetes screening. *Pharm J* 1998; 260: 155.
10. *Practice Guidance on Early Identification of Diabetes by Community Pharmacists*. Royal Pharmaceutical Society of Great Britain – prepared in conjunction with Diabetes UK. September 2001.
11. World Health Organization. *Definition, Diagnosis and Classification of Diabetes Mellitus and its complications (Part 1)*. World Health Organization, Department of Non-communicable Disease Surveillance, Geneva. 1999.
12. Diabetes UK. '*Are you at risk of diabetes? Try this quick test to find out*'. Diabetes UK, 10 Queen Anne Street, London, W1M 0BD.
13. Herman W H, Smith P J, Thompson T J, *et al*. A new sample questionnaire to identify people at increased risk of undiagnosed diabetes. *Diabetes Care* 1995; 18: 382–387.

16

Pharmaceutical assessment of people with diabetes

Diabetes is a life-long condition and the treatment and care required will vary over time. The experience of the quality of care and information provided by health professionals during the first days, weeks and months after diagnosis of diabetes influences the effectiveness of long-term care and subsequent health outcomes for people with diabetes.

In order for people with diabetes to take charge of managing their condition, by making informed choices about their lifestyle and treatment, they need to understand that they are at risk of developing diabetic complications (ketoacidosis or non-ketotic hyperosmolar coma, retinopathy, nephropathy, neuropathy and cardiovascular disease). They also need to be aware of the possible adverse effects of the treatment such as hypoglycaemia with insulin or sulphonylurea therapy.

The main objectives for the management of diabetes mellitus are to:

- minimise the risks of the disease
- minimise the risks of the treatment.

There are various opportunities for pharmacists to carry out an assessment of the needs of a person with diabetes mellitus, the most obvious one being on presentation of a prescription for antihyperglycaemic medication. Other opportunities include requests for information on suitability of OTC products for people with diabetes. It is not possible to provide a standard approach for pharmaceutical assessments that would be appropriate for every situation in which there is an interaction between the pharmacist and people with diabetes. However, pharmacists may find it useful to adapt the checklists outlined below to suit their particular working environment.

Minimising the risks of the disease

The two main principles for 'minimising the risks of the disease' are to encourage the patient to maintain glycaemic control and to adopt a 'healthy' lifestyle (see Management Focus, p. 30). Pharmacists can contribute by providing information on measures for maintaining good glycaemic control and a healthy lifestyle (e.g. diet, exercise, smoking cessation; see Chapters 4 and 5) and by providing information to enable people with diabetes manage 'events' associated with their condition. Events associated with diabetes mellitus include diabetic ketoacidosis, hyperosmolar non-ketotic coma, severe hypoglycaemia, major treatment change (e.g. starting insulin), eye complications, renal complications, 'at-risk' foot, coronary heart disease, stroke, erectile dysfunction or any other new complication.

PHARMACIST CHECKLIST FOR MINIMISING THE RISKS OF THE DISEASE

Complications of the disease

Is the person with diabetes mellitus aware of:

○ The relationship between high blood glucose levels and development of complications such as retinopathy, neuropathy, nephropathy and the diabetic foot?
See Chapter 3, pp. 11–18.

○ The higher risk of cardiovascular disease in people with diabetes?
See Chapter 3, pp. 18–28.

○ The relationship between diet, exercise, antihyperglycaemic medication and blood glucose levels?
See Chapter 6.

○ The reasons for monitoring their blood glucose?
See Chapter 5.

○ The symptoms of hyperglycaemia?
See Chapter 2, p. 5 and Chapter 15, Risk Factors Focus, p. 137.

○ The steps to follow to manage their diabetes when feeling unwell?
See Chapter 4, Management Focus, p. 35.

○ Any other medication they are taking which may impair glucose tolerance or interfere with glucose monitoring tests?
See Chapter 3, Management Focus, p. 29 and Chapter 5, Glucose Monitoring Focuses, pp. 53–55.

Minimising the risks of the treatment

This is an area in which pharmacists can make a significant contribution by utilising their knowledge of medicines and related products. There is evidence of poor adherence to oral antihyperglycaemic drug therapy in people prescribed a combination of oral antihyperglycaemic drug therapy, multiple daily dosage regimens and other co-medications. Simplification of complicated therapeutic drug regimens is a major challenge, but if achieved, it can have a major impact on both the effectiveness of the treatment and the quality of life of people with type 2 diabetes. The incidence of adverse drug reactions can be reduced if simple risk factors associated with complications have been identified and, if possible, eliminated. Risk factors for medication-related adverse events include medication errors. The potential for supply and administration of the wrong type of insulin should be minimised as far as possible by adopting a policy of 'always checking with the patient' that the insulin being supplied is the one they are expecting. There is an increased risk of adverse drug reactions in those with hepatic or renal impairment. The risk of renal disease and drug-induced liver damage is greater in those with diabetes. Elderly patients are also at increased risk. Malnutrition, especially in the elderly in nursing homes, is common. There may be difficulties with timing of meals to coincide with antidiabetic drug treatment. Adverse drug reactions, in relation to diabetes management, may be divided into the following categories:

- Hypoglycaemia with insulin, sulphonylurea or meglitinide treatment.
- Lactic acidosis with metformin treatment.
- Adverse effects with thiazolidinedione (PPAR-γ agonist) treatment.
- Adverse effects due to other concurrent drug therapy.

PHARMACIST CHECKLIST FOR MINIMISING THE RISKS OF THE TREATMENT

Hypoglycaemia with insulin therapy (see pp. 92–93)

Is the person with diabetes mellitus aware of:

○ The symptoms of hypoglycaemia and the action to take in the event of a hypoglycaemic episode occurring?
See Chapter 4, Adverse Effects Focus, p. 37.

○ Any problems with monitoring their blood glucose levels?
See Chapter 5, Glucose Monitoring Focus, p. 49.

○ Any recent changes in the insulin dosage or the type of insulin used?
See Chapter 8, pp. 85–92.

○ Any other prescribed medication that may enhance the hypoglycaemic effect of insulin therapy?
See Chapter 8, pp. 94–97.

○ Recent discontinuation of any prescribed medication that may have impaired glucose tolerance?
See Chapter 3, Management Focus, p. 29.

○ Recent intake or discontinuation of any OTC medicines or complementary medicines that may potentially cause problems?
See Chapter 16 and Adverse Effects Focus, p. 146 and Chapter 6, pp. 63–66.

○ Taking any medication that may interfere with glucose monitoring tests?
See Chapter 5, Glucose Monitoring Focuses, pp. 53–55.

○ The effect on their glycaemic control of varying the insulin injection site?
See Chapter 8, pp. 83–84.

○ The relationship between the timing of the insulin injection and consumption of food?
See Chapter 8, pp. 88–92.

○ The effects of alcohol?
See Chapter 4, p. 42.

○ Their individual response to different types and levels of exercise?
See Chapter 4, pp. 39–41.

**Hypoglycaemia with sulphonylurea or meglitinide therapy
(see pp. 92–93 and p. 130)**

Is the person with diabetes mellitus aware of:

○ The symptoms of hypoglycaemia and the action to take in the event of a hypoglycaemic episode occurring?
See Chapter 4, Adverse Effects Focus, p. 37.

○ Any problems with monitoring their blood glucose levels?
See Chapter 5, Glucose Monitoring Focus, p. 49.

○ The importance of eating regular meals?
See Chapter 4, pp. 35–39.

○ Any recent changes in the sulphonylurea or meglitinide prescribed, or the dosage used?
See Chapter 9, pp. 106–107 and Table 9.1.

○ Any other prescribed medication that may enhance the hypo-glycaemic effect of sulphonylurea or meglitinide therapy?
See Chapter 9, pp. 108–111.

○ Recent discontinuation of any prescribed medication that may have impaired glucose tolerance?
See Chapter 3, Management Focus, p. 29.

○ Recent intake or discontinuation of any OTC medicines or com-plementary medicines that may potentially cause problems?
See Chapter 16 and Adverse Effects Focus, p. 146 and Chapter 6, pp. 63–66.

○ Taking any medication that may interfere with glucose monitoring tests?
See Chapter 5, Glucose Monitoring Focuses, pp. 53–55.

○ The effects of alcohol?
See Chapter 4, p. 42.

○ Their individual response to different types and level of exercise?
See Chapter 4, pp. 39–41.

Lactic acidosis with metformin therapy (see pp. 115–116)

○ Does the person with diabetes have a condition that may induce lactic acidosis with metformin therapy?
See Chapter 10, Adverse Effects Focus, p. 115.

○   Is the person with diabetes taking any other medication that may increase their predisposition to metformin-induced lactic acidosis? *See Chapter 10, pp. 116–117.*

○   Is the person with diabetes aware of the effects of alcohol? *See Chapter 10, p. 116.*

Adverse effects with thiazolidinedione (PPAR-γ-agonist) treatment (see pp. 125–126)

○   Does the person with diabetes know why it is necessary to have regular liver function test? *See Chapter 12, p. 126.*

○   Does the person with diabetes have a history of heart failure? *See Chapter 12, p. 125.*

Adverse effects of other concurrent drug therapy

○   Is the person with diabetes taking any concurrent medication that may potentially cause problems? *See Chapter 3, Management Focuses, pp. 23–26 and p. 29; Chapter 6, pp. 63–66 and Chapter 16, Adverse Effects Focus, pp. 146–147.*

ADVERSE EFFECTS FOCUS

Potential problems with OTC medicines in diabetes

Analgesics. *Aspirin* affects blood glucose (see pp. 96–97, salicylates). Although people with diabetes can take aspirin (see Chapter 3), *paracetamol* or *ibuprofen* may be safer alternatives for occasional use as an analgesic. Chronic use of *ibuprofen* may affect renal function and this may be of significance in elderly patients. *Paracetamol* causes hepatic damage at high doses and may interfere with some home blood glucose monitoring tests (see Glucose Monitoring Focus, p. 53).

Cold and cough remedies. *Pseudoephedrine* may increase blood pressure in diabetic patients. Blood glucose concentrations are affected by parenteral ephedrine. Nasal administration of *pseudoephedrine* does not appear to cause problems in diabetic patients.

continued overleaf

Adverse Effects Focus (continued)

Gastrointestinal system. Gastrointestinal disturbances can be caused by oral antidiabetics, particularly metformin (see p. 116) and acarbose (see p. 120). Antacids are not effective in treating acarbose-induced gastrointestinal disturbances which are dose-dependent.

Antacids. Magnesium hydroxide and *sodium bicarbonate* affect the absorption of sulphonylureas (see pp. 108–109).

H₂-antagonists. Cimetidine inhibits renal excretion of metformin (see p. 117) and can enhance hypoglycaemic effect of *sulphonylureas* (see p. 110).

Antidiarrhoeal preparations. Diarrhoea can upset diabetic control. It is important that reasonable calorific and fluid intake is maintained. *Oral rehydration solutions* are useful as they facilitate fluid uptake. Anti-motility drugs such as *loperamide* may be used. Adsorbants such as *kaolin* are not recommended for acute diarrhoea and may interfere with absorption of food which in turn affects diabetic control. Vomiting can be a symptom of worsening diabetic control (see pp. 33–35).

Anthelmintics. Mebendazole stimulates insulin secretion and therefore can enhance the hypoglycaemic effect of antidiabetic drugs (see p. 96).

Infections. Diabetic patients are not necessarily more prone to infection, but infections of the genitourinary system can be a sign of poor glycaemic control. Genitourinary infections are associated with risk of renal complications. Referral to the GP for evaluation is recommended for recurrent or persistent cystitis or vaginal candidiasis. *Fluconazole* and *miconozole* can enhance the hypoglycaemic effect of sulphonylureas (see Chapter 9). Infections can cause blood glucose control to deteriorate and increase the risk of ketoacidosis or non-ketotic hyperosmolar coma (see pp. 33–35).

Foot care products. People with diabetes are at risk of developing serious foot problems. Therefore, referral to a chiropodist (specialising in dealing with diabetes related foot problems) is recommended for all foot problems, even if they appear to be minor (see pp. 17–18). Keratolytic preparations (e.g. *salicylic acid* ointment) should not be used.

Dietary supplements. *Vitamin C (ascorbic acid)* supplements can produce false results with some urine and ketone testing reagents and also some home blood glucose monitoring tests (see Glucose Monitoring Focus, pp. 54–55).

Sugar content of medicines. See Chapter 6, p. 59.

National Service Framework for Diabetes: Standards 2002

Summary of evidence base for key interventions for management of diabetes mellitus in adults. This summary excludes diabetes in pregnancy and in children.[1]

Level 1: Meta-analyses, systematic reviews of randomised controlled trials or randomised controlled trials

- Individuals at increased risk of developing type 2 diabetes can reduce their risk if they are supported to change their lifestyle by eating a balanced diet, losing weight and increasing their physical activity levels.
- Structured education can improve knowledge, blood glucose control, weight and dietary management, physical activity and psychological well-being, particularly when this is tailored to the needs of the individual and includes skills-based approaches to education.
- Improving blood glucose control reduces the risk of developing the microvascular complications of diabetes in people with both type 1 and type 2 diabetes.
- Improving blood glucose control may reduce the risk of people with diabetes developing cardiovascular disease.
- Controlling raised blood pressure in people with diabetes who have co-existing hypertension reduces their risk of developing both microvascular complications and cardiovascular disease.
- Regular recall and review of people with diabetes can improve the quality of diabetes care and subsequent outcomes for people with diabetes.
- Regular surveillance for diabetic retinopathy in adults with diabetes and early laser treatment of those identified as having sight-threatening retinopathy can reduce the incidence of new visual impairment and blindness in people with diabetes.
- Treatment of people who have microalbuminuria with ACE inhibitors can reduce their rate of progression to diabetic nephropathy.

- Tight blood pressure and blood glucose control in people with diabetic nephropathy can reduce the rate of deterioration in their function, as well as their risk of cardiovascular disease.
- People with diabetes identified as being at increased risk of developing lower-limb complications can reduce this risk by participating in a foot-care programme that provides foot-care education, podiatry and, where required, protective footwear.
- In people with diabetes who develop foot ulceration, prompt intervention can minimise their risk of subsequent disability and amputation.
- People with diabetes who have established cardiovascular disease can benefit from secondary prevention measures already recommended for general population in the National Service Framework for Coronary Heart Disease.
- Administration of intensive insulin therapy to people with diabetes who sustain a heart attack can reduce their risk of death by 30%.

Level 2: Systematic reviews of case-control or cohort studies, or case control or cohort studies

- Follow-up and regular testing of individuals known to be at increased risk of developing diabetes (people who have previously been found to have impaired glucose regulation and women with a history of gestational diabetes) can lead to the earlier diagnosis of diabetes.
- Opportunistic screening of people with multiple risk factors for diabetes can lead to the identification of some individuals with previously undiagnosed diabetes.
- Reducing cholesterol levels in people with diabetes who have raised cholesterol levels may reduce their risk of cardiovascular disease.
- Smoking cessation in people with diabetes who smoke reduces their risk of both cardiovascular disease and microvascular complications.

Level 3: Non-analytic studies, e.g. case reports or case series

- Increased awareness of the symptoms and signs of diabetes among both health professionals and general public can result in earlier identification of people with diabetes.
- Outcomes for people with diabetes following admission to hospital can be improved by better liaison between the diabetes team and ward staff.
- Perioperative outcomes for people with diabetes can be improved by

adherence to locally agreed evidence-based guidelines for the management of people with diabetes during surgical procedures.

Level 4: Expert opinion (in the absence of any of the above)

- The overall prevalence of type 2 diabetes in the population can be reduced by preventing and reducing the prevalence of overweight and obesity and the prevalence of central obesity in the general population, particularly in sub-groups of the population at increased risk of developing diabetes, such as people from minority ethnic communities, by promoting a balanced diet and physical activity.
- Personal care plans can help empower people with diabetes.
- Patient held/accessed records can facilitate self-care.
- The risk and severity of diabetic ketoacidosis can be reduced by the provision of guidance and advice to people with diabetes on how to manage changes in blood glucose control that occur during other illnesses ('sick day' rules).
- Most episodes of hypoglycaemia can be managed in the community, either by the person with diabetes, a relative or carer, their GP or by ambulance personnel.

References

1.   Department of Health. National Service Framework for Diabetes: Standards 2002. www.doh.gov.uk/nsf/diabetes (last accessed November 2002).

Glossary

Acidosis: accumulation of acid or loss of base resulting in a pathologic condition.

Advanced glycation end-products (AGEs): glycation of tissues caused by chronic high levels of blood glucose. Glycation involves chemical condensation of sugar with free amino acid groups. AGEs may be involved in the pathogenesis of diabetic complications such as atherosclerosis and nephropathy.

Apoproteins: constituents of lipoproteins involved in lipoprotein metabolism.

Cholesterol: steroid molecule with a hydrocarbon side chain forming structural components of cell membranes. The majority of the body's cholesterol is synthesised in the liver.

Diabetic acidosis: metabolic acidosis in which the acid–base status shifts towards the acid; produced by accumulation of ketones.

Dyslipidaemia: low levels of high-density lipoprotein (HDL) cholesterol and high levels of triglycerides.

Gluconeogenesis: biosynthesis of glucose molecules from amino acids and fatty acids.

Glycogenesis: biosynthesis of glycogen.

Glycogenolysis: breakdown of glycogen into glucose.

Glycolysis: breakdown of glucose.

High-density lipoprotein (HDL): carriers of plasma cholesterol (carry approximately 20%).

Ketogenesis: formation of ketones.

Lactic acidosis: a metabolic acidosis due to excess lactic acid in the blood; produced by conditions which impair cellular respiration.

Lipogenesis: biosynthesis of fat.

Lipolysis: breakdown of fat.

Lipodystrophy: disturbance of fat metabolism.

Lipogenic: formed or caused by fat.

Lipohypertrophy: hypertrophy of subcutaneous fat caused by lipogenic effects of insulin.

Lipoproteins: particles involved in transport of cholesterol and triglycerides in plasma.

Local Diabetes Services Advisory Groups (LDSAG): local health authority liaison groups usually consisting of healthcare professionals, people with diabetes and their carers.

Low-density lipoproteins (LDL): main carriers of cholesterol between the liver and peripheral tissues.

Metabolic acidosis: a metabolic disturbance due to loss of base or retention of non-carbonic, or fixed (non-volatile), acids.

Proteolysis: breakdown of protein.

Polyol pathway: metabolism of glucose by aldose reductase to produce sorbitol. Excessive metabolism via this pathway can lead to accumulation of sorbitol which causes swelling and tissue damage. Aldose reductase inhibitors have a potential therapeutic use in slowing down progression of neuropathy.

Somogyi effect: rebound hyperglycaemic reaction in the morning in response to low blood glucose concentrations at around 3 a.m. It has been suggested that this effect is due to activation of glucose production by the liver by insulin counter-regulatory hormones (e.g. cortisol, glucagon and adrenaline).

St Vincent Declaration: a consensus document setting out targets for improvement in the quality and duration of life of people with diabetes mellitus. The document resulted from a meeting held at St Vincent, Italy in October 1989 under the auspices of the European sections of the World Health Organization (WHO E) and International Diabetes Federation (IDF E).

Triglycerides: fatty acids condensed onto glycerol; main fuel storage in the body. Source, dietary or synthesised in the liver.

Very-low-density lipoproteins (VLDL): carriers of triglycerides.

Useful resources

Websites

British Heart Foundation's statistics website: www.heartstats.org
Department of Health. www.doh.gov.uk/traveladvice/index.htm
Diabetes UK: www.diabetes.org.uk
Healthtalk: www.healthtalk.com
National Institute for Clinical Excellence clinical guidelines for diabetes management. www.nice.org.uk
American Association of Diabetes Educators: www.aadenet.org
American Diabetes Organization: www.diabetes.org/main
Diabetes Exercise and Sports Association: www.diabetes-exercise.org
International Diabetes Federation: www.idf.org/home/index.cfm?node=1

Journal articles and original papers

Aburuz S M, McElnay J C, Millership J S, *et al*. Factors affecting self-care activities, postprandial plasma glucose and HbA1c in patients with type 2 diabetes. *Int J Pharmacy Practice* 2002; 10 (suppl): R96.

Anonymous. Special feature: New products overview [blood glucose monitoring and insulin delivery devices], Ouch! *Diabetes Update* 2002; Autumn: 23–28.

Bliss E. Diabetes care – an evaluation of a community pharmacy based HbA1c testing service. *Pharm J* 2001; 267: 264–266.

Burrill P. Is self-monitoring of glycaemic control of any value? *Pharm J* 2002; 268: 847–848.

Dixon N. Pharmacists as part of an extended diabetes team. *Pharm J* 2002; 268: 469–470.

Douglas E, Hudson S, Bennie M, *et al*. Pharmaceutical care needs in the primary care management of type 2 diabetes mellitus. BPC 2000 Pharmacy Practice Research paper. *Pharm J* 2000; 265: R6.

Gill G V, Redmond S. Insulin treatment, time-zones and air travel. A survey of current advice from British diabetic clinics. *Diabet Med* 1993; 10: 764–767.

McClean M T, McElnay J C, Andrews J. The importance of patient education and patient involvement in the treatment of diabetes. BPC 2000 Pharmacy Practice Research paper. *Pharm J* 2000; 265: R20.

Montopoli T. Diabetes care. How to handle common questions from patients with diabetes. *Pharm Pract* 1998; 14: 62–71.

Simmonds R. Diabetes screening and a role for the High Street pharmacist. *Mod Diabetes Management* 2002; 3: 6–7.

Tadros L, Barnes E, Ledger-Scott M. Hospital pharmacists' role in type 2 diabetes management. *Int J Pharmacy Practice* 2002; 10 (suppl): R87.

Guidelines

Diabetes UK and Royal Pharmaceutical Society of GB. *Care Recommendation: Early Identification of Diabetes for Community Pharmacists.* August 2001.

Royal Pharmaceutical Society of GB Diabetes Task Force. *Practice Guidance for Community Pharmacists on the Care of People with Diabetes*, 2nd edition. February 2001.

National Institute for Clinical Excellence. *Managing Blood Pressure and Blood Lipid Levels. A Guide for Adults with Type 2 Diabetes.* October 2002.

Department of Health. *National Service Framework for Diabetes: Standards 2002.*

Diabetes UK. *Recommendations for Management of Diabetes in Primary Care.* Report. October 2000.

Greenhalgh P M. *Shared Care for Diabetes; a Systematic Review.* Royal College of General Practitioners Occasional Paper No. 67. London 1994.

Books

Hillson R. *Diabetes. A New Guide.* Positive Health Guides. Chapter 15. The diabetes team and the diabetes service. London: Optima, 1992.

Mackinnon M. *Providing Diabetes Care in General Practice*, 2nd edition. London: Class Publishing, 1995. Chapter 1. Responsibilities of those involved in the provision of diabetes care; Chapter 13. Education for self management.

Shillitoe R. *Counselling People with Diabetes.* Communication and Counselling in Health Care Series. BPS Books (The British Psychological Society), 1994.

Watkins P J. *ABC of Diabetes*, 4th edition. Chapter 18. Diabetes and pregnancy; Chapter 19. Organisation of diabetes care including shared care schemes. BMJ Publishing Group, 1998.

Watkins P J, Drury P L, Howell S L. *Diabetes and its Management*, 5th edition. Chapter 11. Diabetic emergencies: ketoacidosis, non-ketotic states and management during surgery; Chapter 20. Diabetes in children and adolescents. Oxford: Blackwell Scientific Publications, 1996.

Index

Entries in *italic* type refer to brand names. Page numbers in **bold** type refer to entries in boxes, figures and tables.